Kurt Tittel

Muscle Slings in Sport

Analysing Movements in Various Disciplines from a Functional-Anatomical Point of View

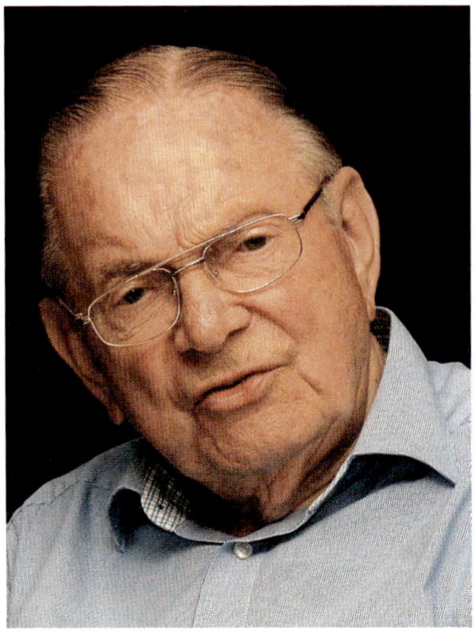

© private

Prof. em. Dr. med. Dr. h. c. Kurt Tittel

Emeritus Professor and former Chairman of the Department of Functional Anatomy of the University of Halle and of the Hochschule für Körperkultur (Institute of Physical Culture) in Leipzig.

Former Chairman of the Department of Sports Medicine of the Academy for continuous professional development in Berlin-Lichtenberg.

This textbook describes the activity of muscle slings in professional athletes and is, in part, based on material presented in the 15th edition of the German textbook "Beschreibende und funktionelle Anatomie" (descriptive and functional anatomy), by K. Tittel with the assistance of E. Seidel, published by KIENER Verlag, Munich 2012.

International honours

Philip-Noel Baker Research Price of the International Council of Sport Science and Physical Education (CIEPSS) for scientific contributions in the field of Sports-Anthropometry (1974)

Distinguished Service Award of the United States Sports Academy for noteworthy contributions to International Sport (1984)

Honorary Prize of the International Olympic Committee in appreciation of outstanding services in the field of Sports Medicine (1989)

Honorary-Membership of the Hungarian Sports Medical-Association (1984)

Honorary-Membership of the Czechoslowakian Purkinje-Association (1984)

Gold medal of the International Federation of Sports Medicine (FIMS) and appointment as FIMS Fellow (2002)

Kurt Tittel

Muscle Slings in Sport

Analysing Movements in Various Disciplines from a Functional-Anatomical Point of View

Translation by Paul Crichton and Christl Kiener

1st edition, 118 illustrations

KIENER PRESS Munich 2015

Working title of the unpublished manuscript:
"Analyse von Bewegungsabläufen im Sport aus funktionell-anatomischer Sicht"
(Analysis of sequences of movements in sport from a functional anatomical point of view)

Notice
Neither the publisher nor the author assumes any responsibility for any loss or injury and/or damage to persons arising out of or related to any use of the material contained in this book. It is the responsibility of the treating practitioner, relying on independent expertise and knowledge of the patient, to determine the best treatment and method of application for the patient.

British Library Cataloguing in Publication Data
A catalogue record of this book is available from the British Library (www.bl.uk)
Library of the Congress Cataloguing in Publication Data
A catalogue record for this book is available from the Library of the Congress (www.loc.gov)
Deutsche Nationalbibliothek/Bayerische Staatsbibliothek in Publication Data
A catalogue record of this book is available from the Deutsche Nationalbibliothek (www.d-nb.de) and **Bayerische Staatsbibliothek** (www.bsb-muenchen.de).

1st edition 2015
KIENER Press, Munich

Translation: Paul Crichton, London; Christl Kiener, München
Editing: Christl Kiener, München
Illustrations/Photos: Kurt Opitz, Leipzig; Henriette Rintelen, Velbert
Layout design: Kadja Gericke, Arnstorf
Cover design: SpieszDesign, Neu-Ulm
Cover illustration: Kurt Opitz, Leipzig
Printing and binding: Drukarnia Dimograf, Bielsko-Biała/Poland

ISBN 978-3-943324-41-9

www.kiener-press.com

Preface

Movement in every-day life and in sport shows that the functional and structural adaptation of the active and passive motor system to physical strain of variable duration and intensity is a precondition of high physical performance. It should be based on a well-balanced and well-trained interplay of the muscular agonists and antagonists responsible for dynamic and static movements. This interplay becomes all the more necessary for the planning and implementation of prophylaxis, training methodology and physiotherapy, when one considers the increasing physical specialization and the inappropriate strain which is sometimes put on muscles, both at work and particularly in sport. To achieve this aim, it is not primarily the size or power of a single muscle, however well developed, which is important, but rather the way it can function optimally in the context of movements of a part or of the whole of the body, when it is combined with other agonists and antagonists to form "muscle slings", which operate as a functional unit. In this way stable muscle-joint relationships are established, which guarantee that the movement and support system of our body can withstand great stress.

This is what the numerous and interesting sequences of movements, carried out by female and male athletes in various types of sport, are intended to demonstrate. At the same time the reader will learn about the important part played by a functional-anatomical approach to the motor system in every-day life and practice. The content is intended to meet the needs of sports training, physio- and sports therapy, and rehabilitation following injuries. The text is superbly complemented by the unique three-part illustrations created by the artist, Kurt Opitz.

This book has been written especially for sports students, and for physio-, sport- and ergo-therapeutic students, as well as for trainers and sports physicians in continuous professional development. The author was actively involved in anatomy and sports medicine for almost four decades, and had medical responsibility for professional athletes at a national and international level, and was thus in continuous contact with the practical aspects of sport. He hopes that, with this book, he can give the reader some new and interesting insights and stimulating ideas for his or her own work.

I wish to give special thanks to KIENER Press in Munich and to the translators for their professional and committed support and reliable cooperation.

Kurt Tittel
Leipzig, June 2015

Table of Contents

1

Analysis of sequences of movements in sport from a functional-anatomical point of view

1.1 Adaptability of the motor system as a process and outcome

For the analysis of sequences of movements in sport from a functional-anatomical point of view it is necessary to have a basic knowledge of the structure and function of the motor system, of the interconnection between its main components and of their functional and structural, quantitative and qualitative biological adaptability to physical stress of varying duration and intensity.

Such progressive stress-, age- and gender-dependent functional and structurally enhanced performance of the motor system is achieved on the basis of an epigenetically predetermined regulatory system and must repeatedly be activated to meet the demands made on it. This **enhanced performance of the motor system** has stimulated scientific and practical interest in the increasing of the weight-bearing capacity and recovery capability of the active and passive motor system in sport. The initial results have influenced very significantly the nature of training and sports medicine as well as the prophylaxis, therapy and rehabilitation of injuries and the effects of abnormal stress.

In this connection we should consider the following facts:

- the considerable increase in the cross-section of the tendons with an increase of the tensile strength of the tendon fibrils
- the reversible increase in the thickness (hypertrophy) of the hyaline joint cartilage after endurance training
- the dynamic plasticity of the cancellous structure (spongiosa) inside the bone
- the increase of the thickness (between 5 % and 20 %) and the bone mineral density of the hard, lamellar bone surface (corticalis)
- the triangular cross-section of the tibia, the ulna, and the lower humerus and femur
- the increase in (and lordosis of) the surface area of the vertebrae and the increase in the resistance to compression of the lower thoracic and all the lumbar vertebrae after a longer period of maximal strength training (fig. 1) and

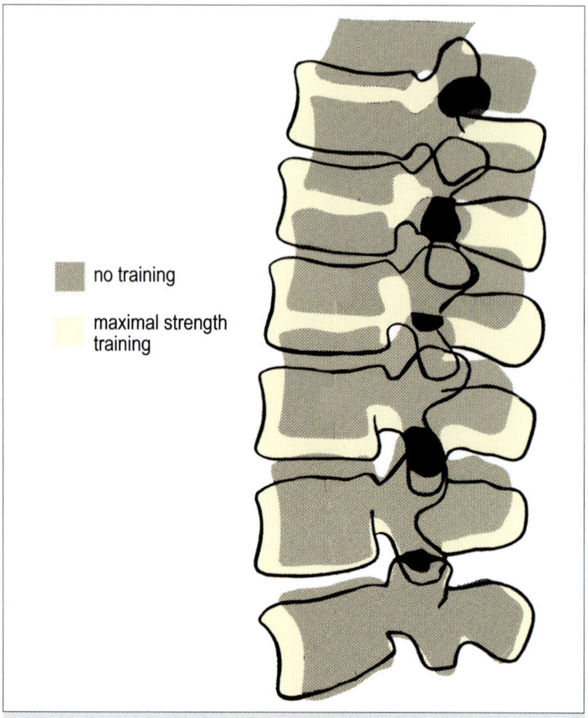

Fig. 1 The increase in (and lordosis of) the surface area of the lower thoracic and all the lumbar vertebrae in athletes after a longer period of maximal strength training.

- the specific adaptation of the skeletal muscles: reversible functional and structural hypertrophy of the types of muscle fibres which are primarily affected by power training (i.e. increase in muscle mass but not in the number of muscle fibres), functional enlargement of the capillary system (fig. 2) as well as an increase in the number and surface area of the mitochondria, which supply energy after endurance training.

These macroscopic and submicroscopic as well as biochemically detectable **functional and structural tissue reactions** are specific to demands made by regular, intensive and intermittent physical stress, make strain and subsequent relaxation necessary and must always be considered in an analysis of sequences of movements in sport. **These reactions increase sports performance and exercise tolerance, and accelerate the recovery processes of the organism.**

1.2 Form, structure and function

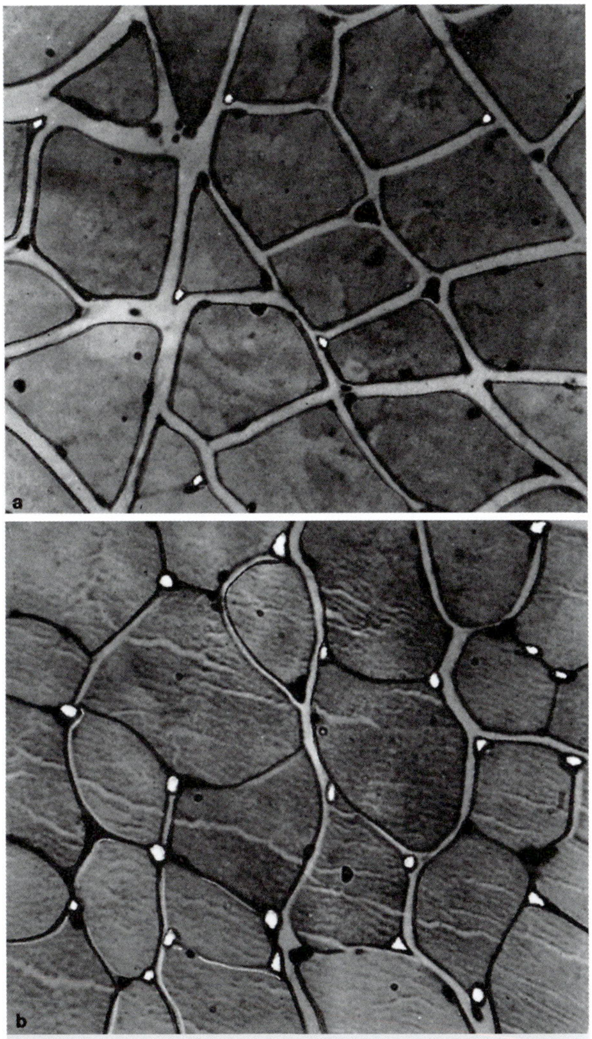

Fig. 2 Capillarisation of an untrained skeletal muscle (a) and one which has undergone endurance training (b) in cross-section; iron haematoxylin dye. 500:1.

Anatomy nowadays is no longer limited to observations made from the dissection of dead material. It is increasingly **focussed on life, on active functioning which is orientated towards practical needs.** Furthermore anatomical knowledge is examined on living organisms (also in animal experiments) in order to gain very detailed information about the interrelationship between organisms and the environment, between the form, the structure of an organ and its function which constantly influence one another. This can be done, for example, by analysing microscopically living muscle tissue obtained by biopsy. The form, structure and function of an individual person must therefore always be considered macroscopically, microscopically and at a molecular level, as **two sides of the same coin.** We should bear in mind that all living things and their functions are linked to organic structures which however represent mere snapshots, mere reactions of the constantly changing organism to the corresponding demands.

! In this connection it is interesting to note that the adaptation of tissue to a stimulus can not only be quantitative, but also qualitative as a qualitatively new tissue can develop. Form, structure and function (mechanical strain) constitute a living unit, which disintegrates only in death.

If you look at a skeleton you see that every bone can only be understood as **part of a whole.** This applies both to the large and long femur with its slightly anterior curvature or the tibia with its triangular cross-section.

- The transverse axis at the level of the knee joint, for example, is shifted posteriorly by the anterior convex curvature of the femur (fig. 3). As a result there is an increase in stability and a significant degree of flexion of the lower leg against the thigh becomes possible, so that one can sit comfortably with the buttocks on the heels from a kneeling position – which children can do much better than adults.
- Although a column is the most suitable and most economical weight-bearer with regard to material

usage, the tibia always has a triangular shape even when subjected to great pressure and traction forces which are brought about by the extensor muscles of the foot. If these are paralysed or atrophied in early adulthood, then the tibia acquires a more circular and less resilient cross-section.

These two examples show clearly that the long tubular bones resist in an optimal way the dangerous flexion stresses (for example spiral stress in slalom), not only because of their cross-sectional shape but also because of the longitudinal curvature of their shaft (fig. 3), and because of the muscular and ligamental traction belt. Thus they are characterized by a **"functional shape".** Their rough form and inner structure are perfectly suited to bear great axial intermittent pressure-stresses with a minimum amount of material. This applies also to the vertebrae. **There is hardly an organ** – this generalization is perfectly justified after what has already been said – **which does not acquire its functional structure from the whole.** The same applies to sequences of movements which – however simple they may seem – always involve several parts of the body, albeit to differing degrees.

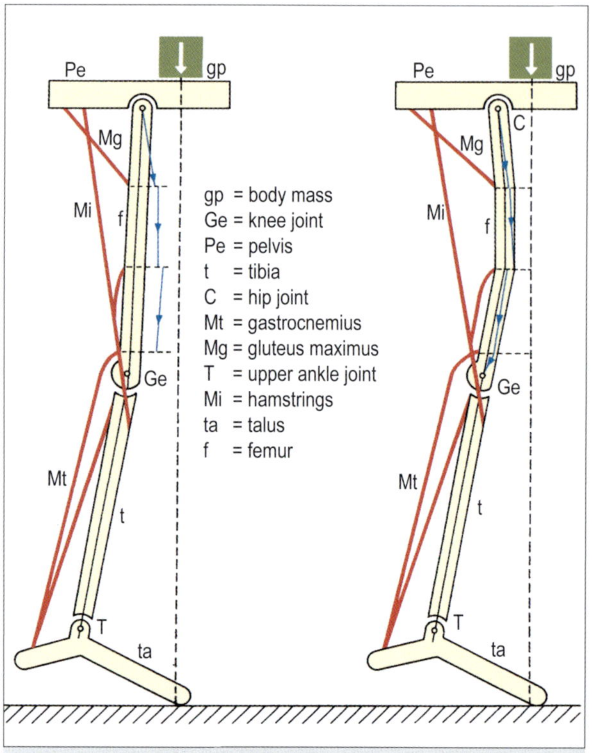

Fig. 3 Adaptation of the shape of the longitudinal axis of the femur to flexion stress. While the illustration on the left shows the position of the stress forces (= arrows), when the femur has just been adducted, the diagram on the right shows that, when the femur is bent to a certain degree, the directions of the force lines of the stress forces in the individual sections come much closer to the vertical axis of the bone, and this results in a significant reduction of the flexion load.

1.3 Open and closed joint systems

In his study of the various movements and their articular connections Baeyer (1924) was the first to coin the functional term "kinematic joint system", instead of an ordinary, anatomically self-contained joint. He was no longer satisfied with the idea that there is a series of limbs which are connected to each other by joints. Moreover he realized that, depending on the kind of movement, different parts of our body come into close contact with forces which lie beyond the body, and this takes place in chain-like processes.

Kinematic joint systems have either a free final link (they are **"open"**), which makes isolated movements possible, which are relatively independent of one another, or they are – and this applies to most movements – **"closed"** at their finishing points by some resistance (for example sports equipment and the ground). Only in this way – among other things as a result of the remote effect of the muscles on joints with which they are not connected – is a firm control of a movement made possible.

The principle of open and closed systems is also

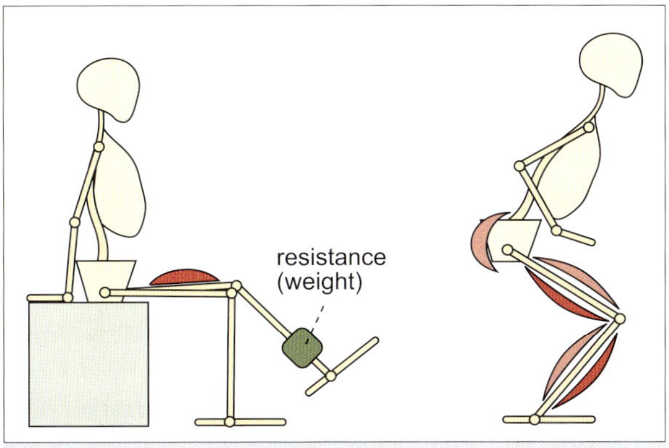

Fig. 4 Open and closed movement system (treatment of a knee joint injury).

used in therapy (movement is therapy). In a clinical setting, relief of strain or partial relief is often necessary and cannot be realised in closed chains. For this reason exercise and training at the beginning of movement therapy must be carried out in an „open" system, and can then be changed to a „closed" system as soon as adequate functionality has been achieved (fig. 4).

A **"closed"** movement chain in sport, for example when one is sitting on a bicycle, consists of **left** upper arm → lower arm → hand → handle bar → **right** hand → lower arm → upper arm → shoulder blade → scapular muscles → spine → **left** scapular muscles → shoulder blade.

An example from sport: in throwing and pushing, the height and the angle of the throw can be optimized – in throwing the discus and the javelin depending on the aerodynamic characteristics of the equipment and the air resistance. On the other hand, the velocity of the throw, which depends on the degree of the acceleration impulse, is the decisive factor for performance. The work done by the body when throwing the javelin, when throwing the discus and when putting the shot is directed **against two kinds of resistance:** the sports equipment and the ground (tartan track or throwing circle) (fig. 5). In both these kinds of resistance the kinetic joint system is "closed". It is opened by the acceleration impulse resulting from the **movement of the whole body,** which is transferred to the javelin, the discus or the shot. The counter-effect, the **"recoil"**, also described as the "reaction force of the ground" is

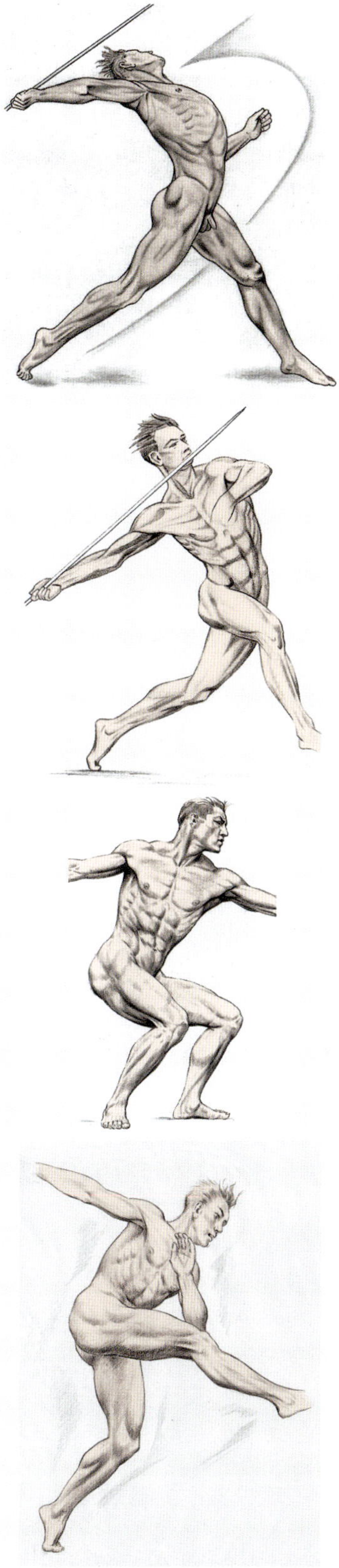

Fig. 5 Throwing the javelin, throwing the discus and kicking the ball are typical examples of whole-body movements, which are closed at their finishing points.

absorbed by the more or less firm ground. This means that forces which exert an effect during the throw and the putting of the shot, but also when walking, running, jumping or climbing (stairs), are not only directed forwards or upwards, but bring their influence to bear down on the ground or the stairs when the heel touches down. The **reaction force of the ground** achieves maximal levels (about 130 % of body weight) and the heel is lifted with about 110 % of body weight. Forces also arise from the ground depending on its properties – which enables the muscles involved in the movement to develop their full power.

Glasgow and Müller (1955) came to the following conclusion in their experiments on walking on different surfaces:

> *"The constant when walking on an even surface in the laboratory is 0.5 cal per m of the distance walked and kg body mass, and it increases by 20 % when walking on a street with the kind of heavy shoes usually worn on a farm, by 40 % on a grassy path, by 70 % on a stubble field or in a potato furrow and by 90 % to 170 % on a freshly ploughed field, depending on its condition."*

Payr (1932) coined the term "kinetic chain", by which he meant:

> *"... the totality of all organs and organic systems and their performance, which provide the significant energy for the voluntary movements of parts of the body, transfer it and bring about the mechanical effects in the target organs, but also provide information about the resulting change of posture, its effect on the amount of power required and the new status quo, and bring about the appropriate physical reaction."*

Payr concluded that every lesion of a link in the chain inevitably causes a disruption of the whole chain.

Further studies, including the work and ideas of Benninghoff (1975), Hoepke (1979), Pauwels (1965) and Braus (1956) were among the **first landmark publications in anatomy which made special reference to functional connections.** This applies inspite of the fact that some of the above-mentioned authors confined themselves partially to local phenomena, and formulated theories which did not always meet the required standard of proof. This also applies, for example, to the hypotheses of the Weber brothers about the forward movement of the leg without muscular power which was disproved shortly afterwards by Duchenne and Fischer.

This was the the starting point, over 50 years ago, for the author and his co-workers to study the chain-like behaviour by **analysing the sequences of movements** of the active and passive motor system **in sport.** We were interested in the interplay between "agonists" and "antagonists" in dynamic and static movements of varying duration and intensity, and in their functional as well as structural effects on the large joints, on the tendinous and ligamental system, as well as on the hyaline and connective tissue, namely cartilage and bone. The results which we achieved were closely linked to the state of theoretical knowledge and the requirements of medical studies and future professional practice. The visual functional-anatomical presentation of the living body was always based on the concept of **the whole body in movement.**

1.4 The cooperation between muscle groups which form muscle slings

We called the muscles which unite (funcitonally) in a concerted action **"muscle slings"**, a term which has been widely used in the theory and practice of sport and sports medicine. This also applies to the connective tissue sheaths, the aponeuroses (fascia) which give protection to, and supply the origin and insertion points for the individual muscles, as well as for groups of muscles. They extend over the whole body and secure the change of shape and mobility in muscle contraction.

With the term "muscle slings" the reader can see that it is not a single muscle, however well-developed it may be, but **only the close functional connection of the muscles** which do most of the work. They are well attuned to each other and **guarantee the precise, powerful, economical and at the same time aesthetic sequence of movements.** The reader will notice that the effect of a muscle is not confined to the immediately adjacent joint. This fact is important, not only for increasing performance in sport but also for the prevention, therapy and rehabilitation of injuries and the consequences of inappropriate stress.

The temporary use, the strength of the contraction as well as the power capacity of the muscles acting synergistically and antagonistically in slings, and their involvement in sequences of movements in a particular sport, can be determined with the help of simultaneous telemetric surface **electromyography** (EMG). With this method it is possible to detect and record the size and the sum of the electrical action-potential differences, which arise as a result of the excitation of the muscle cells in voluntary muscle activity, by means of electrodes on the skin surface. In isometric, concentric and excentric muscle contraction there is a linear relationship between the total electrical activity of the muscle and the power it develops.

In the following chapters it is not so much the function of this or that muscle which will be elucidated but rather the function it fulfils within a higher holistic system, the muscle sling. Studying a sequence of movements in sport in this way, from the perspective of functional anatomy, undoubtedly requires enthusiasm as it requires time-consuming observations and experiments. Even apparently very simple movements can be puzzling when they are analyzed and when practical conclusions are drawn, especially as functional combinations of muscles and their **interplay in "open" and "closed" chains** are varied and change from moment to moment. This can be seen, for example, in the co-contraction of the omohyoideus muscle when someone is wringing out a wet cloth or squeezing a sponge.

! The previous assumption that every muscle has only one specific task depending on its points of origin and insertion is therefore only partly correct. Its function is largely determined by the particular combination of groups of muscles with the enclosed bones, joints and fascia involved, and is subject to frequent changes when one takes into account the different and often opposing functions which one and the same muscle fulfills in open or closed joint chains.

An example of this is the myokinesiographic studies carried out by Scherb (1952) on the mode of contraction of individual muscles when a somebody is walking on a treadmill. These studies have been refined in recent decades with the help of more appropriate investigations (for example by measuring ground pressure and by electromyography). An important result of Scherb's studies is that the following **muscles are involved in the maintenance of the support and active pushing-off phase of the walking and running cycle** (61 % of the time; fig. 6):

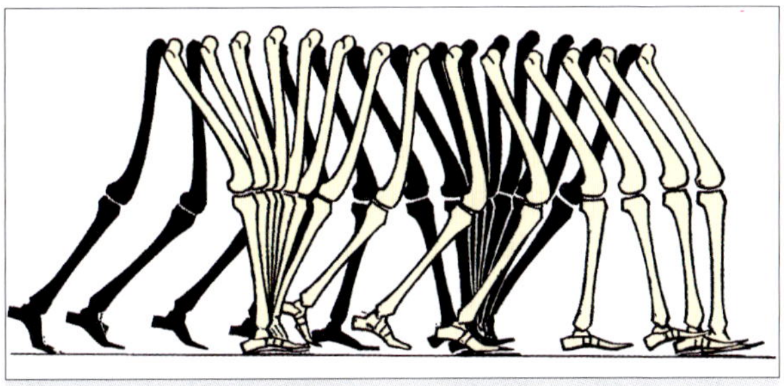

Fig. 6 The leg in the sagittal plane has the function of weight-bearing in the standing position and of pushing the body forward when walking. Each leg has a swing phase and a touching-down phase. This is subdivided into a phase of mere support and a phase of active pushing.

2

Applied anatomy in sport

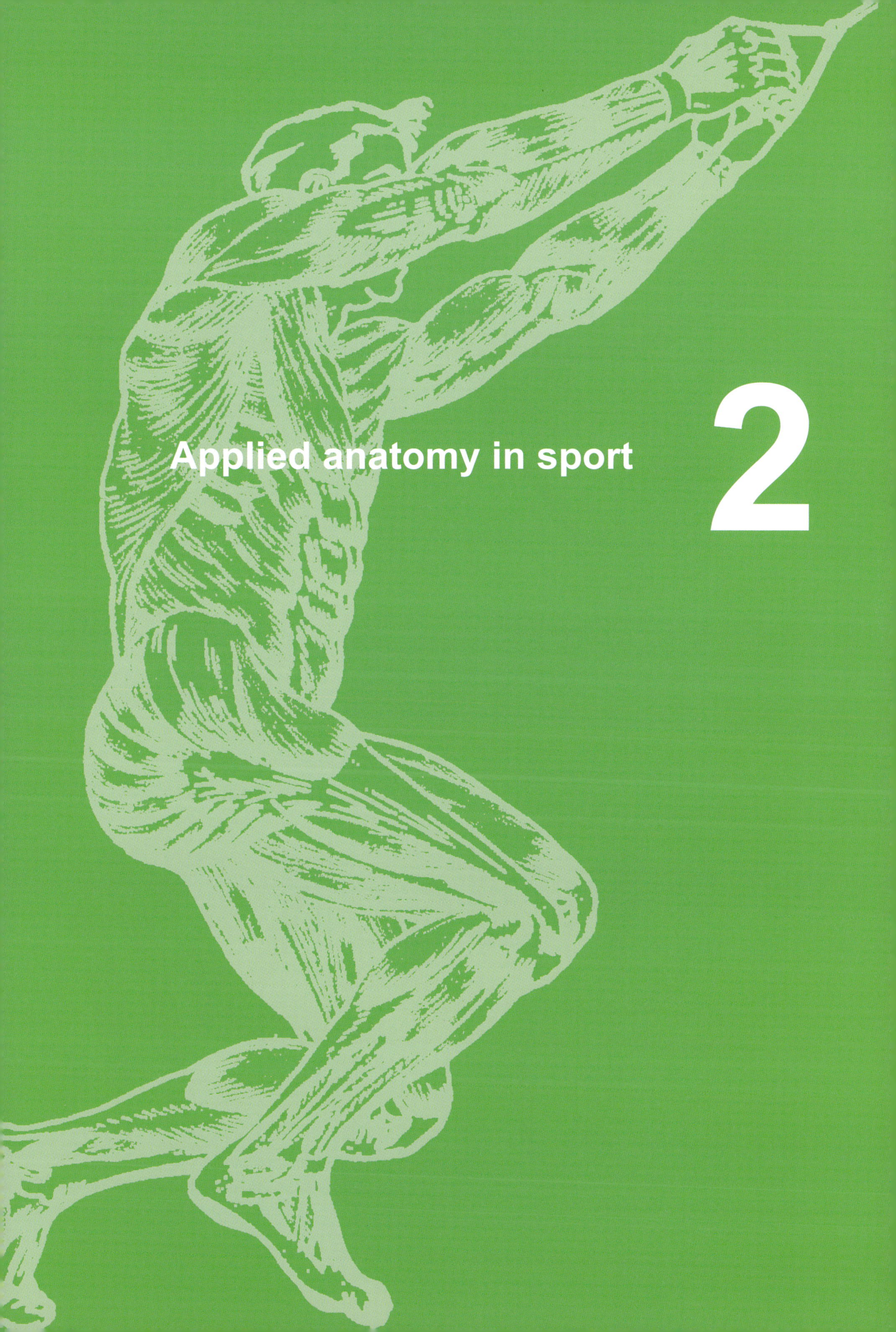

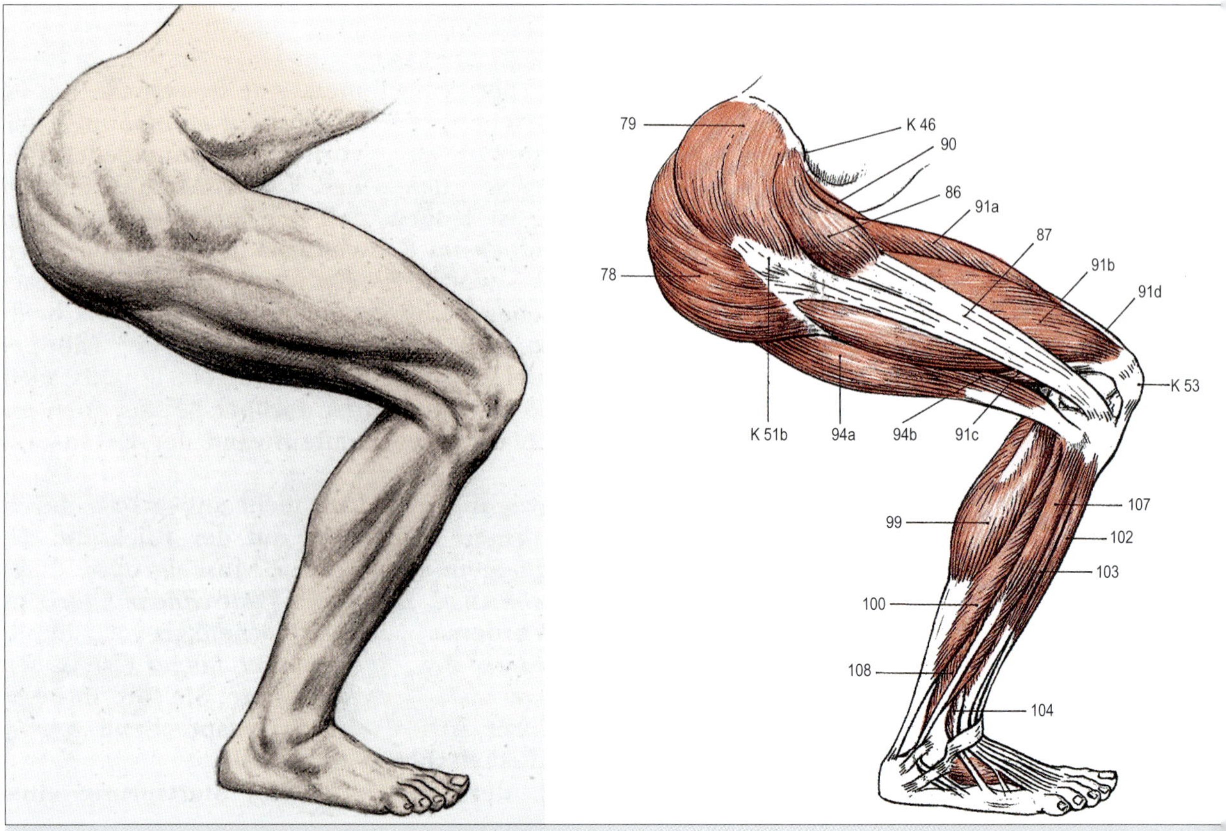

Fig. 15 Basic movement for the illustration of the extensor sling in the lower extremity. One can see in particular the broad reinforcing strand of the fascia lata, the Maissiat band (tractus iliotibialis).

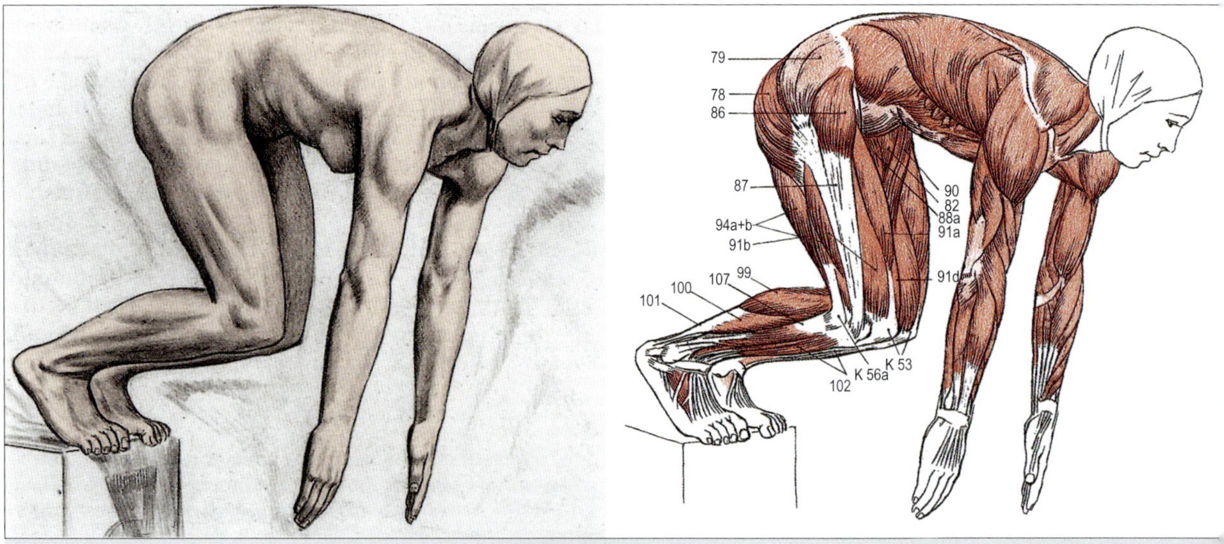

Fig. 16 Extensor sling in the lower extremity of a breast-stroke swimmer during the initial jump from the block. In addition to the conventio way of starting, nowadays the so-called "grip start" is used more frequently. In this case the hands are held on on the front edge of the bloc and then push away and thus support the jump after the starting signal.

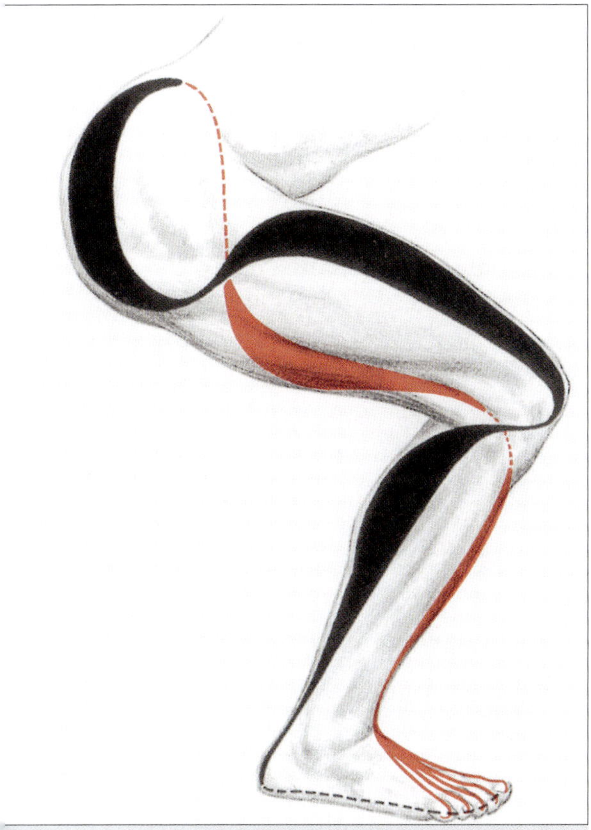

Muscles Fig. 15 and Fig. 16

78 Gluteus maximus
79 Gluteus medius
82 Pectineus
86 Tensor fasciae latae
87 Tractus iliotibialis
88a Adductor longus
90 Sartorius
91a Rectus femoris
91b Vastus lateralis
91c Vastus medialis
91d Vastus intermedius
94a Biceps femoris, caput longum
94b Biceps femoris, caput breve
99 Gastrocnemius
100 Soleus
101 Tendo calcaneus
102 Tibialis anterior
103 Extensor digitorum longus
104 Extensor digitorum brevis
107 Fibularis longus
108 Fibularis brevis

K46 Spina iliaca anterior superior
K51b Trochanter major
K53 Patella
K56a Caput fibulae
K53 Patella

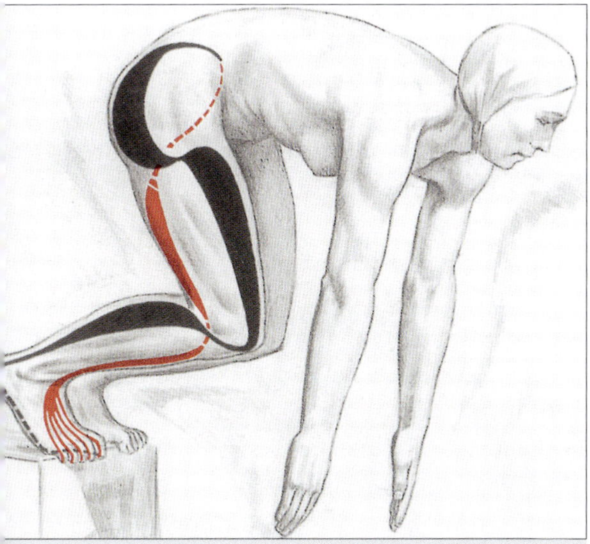

2.1 Extensor slings of the lower extremity

After these preliminary remarks we examine, for a very simple basic movement – the position of the leg at the hip, knee and ankle joint at the beginning of a jump – **which muscles are active for the extension of these joints** (fig. 15). As a preparatory exercise (initial movement) the centre of gravity is lowered by bending the trunk towards the thigh at the hip joint, the thigh towards the lower leg at the knee joint and finally the lower leg towards the foot at the ankle joint. In addition there is, as can be observed with a **swimmer** during her initial dive (fig. 16), a lifting of the foot at the metatarsal balls of the foot. At the same time there is a more or less obvious lifting of the heels from the ground.

After this preparation the relevant extension muscles of the lower extremity are brought into an optimal state of tension and the joints mentioned above into an angular position from which the desired sequence of movements can easily be carried out. A jump can never be executed from a position of extreme extension of the lower extremity because the extensors are already contracted in this position and cannot perform any additional work.

The principle of transfering certain muscles groups from a powerful contraction into a state of extension can be found again and again in many sequences of movements, because **muscles can be optimally shortened only from a position of a well-defined initial position of extension.** This is only possible with a targeted training of the extension capacity of the muscles (with stretching programmes). Some of the starting positions in different sport disciplines have been changed for this reason over time and these changes were associated with the required performance. In this context we should mention the introduction of the crouch start for short-distance runners as well as the varying starting positions of fencers, depending on the duelling sword (épée) and the type of fencing.

In order to make the expected performance of the strong extensor muscles of the lower extremity as efficient as possible, it is necessary to take into consideration that **the centre of gravity of the body** is not shifted too far downwards in the initial movement before the jump. A very strong flexion of the lower extremity uses up part of the strength necessary for the raising of body from a low squatting position. It is therefore advisable to perform a jump from a medium flexion of the knee.

One can easily draw conclusions about the muscles which are needed for the **process of extension** from the **distinctive shape of the surface of the lower extremity** (fig. 15 and 16)**,** as can be observed in well-trained athletes:

- One can identify the strong **gluteus maximus,** which also has an influence on the knee joint via the Maissiat band (by extending the lower leg);
- the **quadriceps femoris** and the **gastrocnemius** together with the **soleus** which bulges outwards from underneath it.

All these muscles with their more or less coarse muscle bundles can be seen and palpated through the skin.

We should first of all look at fig. 15 and the course of the muscles indicated, which are united in a (black) sling extending from the heel to the iliac crest. The contraction of their fibres leads to a **powerful extension of the three joints,** up to this point flexed, and the resistance which these muscles encounter on the solid base leads to a lifting of the body from the ground – a movement which Borelli (1608–1679) in his book *"De motu animalium"* compared to the rapid release of a previously compressed elastic spring.

As a condition of a powerful initial jump the ground (cinder or tartan track, starting blocks in swimming stadiums or the ground), must provide sufficient resistance, in other words must be sufficiently firm.

The **extension movement is however not unlimited.** This is prevented by

- the ischiocrural muscles at the back of the thigh:
  - the biceps femoris,
  - the semitendinosus and semimembranosus muscles and
- the anterior muscles of the lower leg:
  - the tibialis anterior,
  - the extensor hallucis longus and
  - the extensor digitorum longus.

These muscles are shown in a second, weaker (in terms of its performance), red muscle sling.

The conventional start of a swimmer from her block (fig. 16) gives us the opportunity to apply what we have learnt from the basic movement directly to sequences of movements in sport. It should be mentioned that of course at the moment of the initial jump which is shown in the illustration, numerous more or less large powerful muscles are active, for instance the abdominal and dorsal muscles, as well as muscles which have above all holding and supportive functions to maintain an optimal position in the water or which are responsible for forward movement during swimming.

For the time being the only thing of interest is **the cooperation of those muscles which have to do the main work for the initial jump,** i.e.

the extensors of the lower extremity which are combined to form the sling with which we are already familiar. Their tension beneath the skin of the swimmer who is about to jump can be seen in a naturalistic illustration of the sequence of movements (fig. 16) whereas the relief of the trunk and the upper extremities looks rather contourless. The spring-like character of the muscles responsible for the start which is visible even on the skin surface, gives the body great acceleration.

The muscle illustration enables us to check the extent to which our knowledge of the muscles illustrated has been consolidated. This also applies to all the following sequences of movements. Only then should we study the slings represented (and should follow the questions listed above).

The central role of the spinal column in dynamic and static sequences of movements

Structure, function, resilience, weight-bearing capacity

Before we go on to the chapter on the functioning of "extensor slings" (and their corresponding antagonists) in varyious sport disciplines, we shall now discuss in detail the rig-like structure of the **spinal muscles,** because its central role and integration in the athletic movement sequences **are of fundamental importance.**

The **spinal column** (columna vertebralis) in humans consists of 7 cervical, 12 thoracic and 5 lumbar vertebrae, as well as of the sacral and coccygeal bones. It has static and dynamic functions, by giving the body a stable, mobile and elastic support, and by holding up the head, the trunk and the upper extremities, which together make up two-thirds of the total body mass. It also absorbs and transfers the shocks caused by walking and jumping, and it encloses and protects the spinal cord (medulla spinalis) and the roots of the spinal nerves (nervi spinales). The sagittal and transverse bony extensions of the spinal column offer the muscles points of origin and insertion. Thus the spinal column

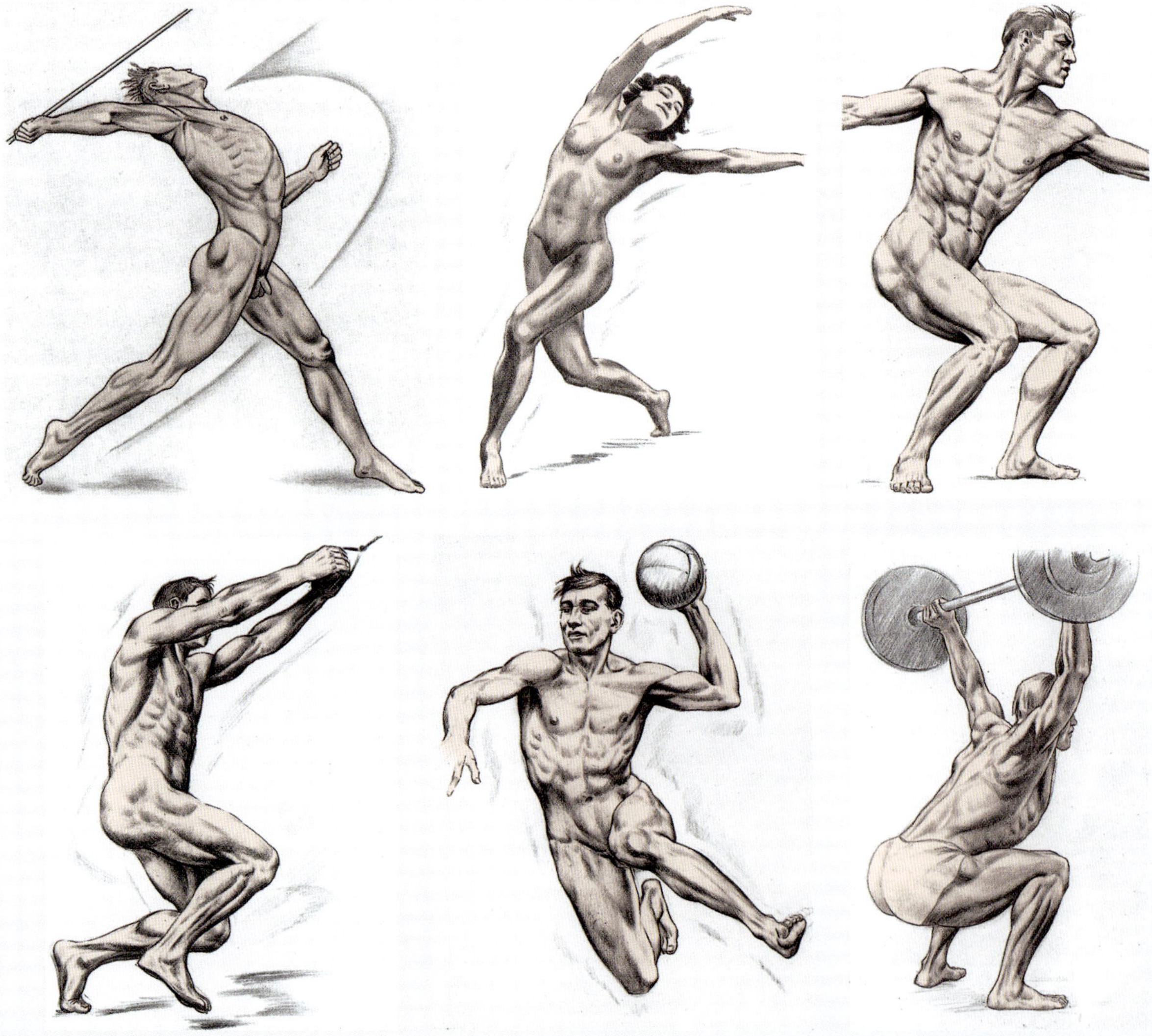

Fig. 17 Movements that require a fully functional spinal column which can also bear larger loads, such as is required for weight lifting.

meets the requirement of being both **as stable as possible and as flexible as necessary.** This raises the question of its ability to tolerate an increase and decrease of stress or load.

The trunk and the spinal column achieve the necessary stability and mobility, due to the functional combination and the well-organized interplay of 133 joints, 224 ligaments and 143 individual muscles in total. These muscles make up 34 % of the entire muscle mass of our body, which consists of 424 muscles.

Sequences of movements such as throwing the javelin, by increasing the lordosis of the entire spinal column (to give the trunk and the muscles the "tension for drawing the bow" required for the throw), or rhythmical gymnastics with pronounced overstretching of the lumbo-sacral transition, or throwing the discus and the hammer with forceful twisting of the trunk and the jump shot in indoor handball – all these movements require a fully functional spinal column, which can also bear larger loads, such as is required for weight lifting (fig. 17).

How does the central axial skeleton, using its functional and anatomical structure, perform these tasks?

The upper 24 vertebrae are slightly mobile against each other due to paired intervertebral joints, and show in their entirety characteristic curvatures in the median and sagittal planes.

These curvatures are formed in the course of the first years of life due to increasing functional strain on this central skeletal axis: a cervical lordosis, a thoracic kyphosis and a lumbar lordosis develop. These are called **physiological spinal curvatures** (fig. 18). As a result of the curvatures acquired with the development of the upright gait the body's vertical axis becomes more resistent to flexion, which reduces the need for muscle activity that would otherwise be necessary to maintain the body's balance, and becomes capable of balancing the trunk and head when standing, walking or jumping. They protect the brain, the spinal cord and other sensitive internal organs from life-threatening lesions caused by pressure and shearing loads.

How great can these pressure or shearing loads be?

The maximal axial pressures tolerated by the vertebrae and intervertebral discs (disci intervertebrales) in a physiologically curved spinal column are:

- in the cervical spine: 54.9 N/cm^2 = 5.5 mPa
- in the thoracic spine: 113.8 N/cm^2 = 11.4 mPa and
- in the lumbar spine: 60.8 N/cm^2 = 6.1 mPa.

This applies, provided that there is strong muscular and ligamental protection of the central axial skeleton. If this is not the case, then the values mentioned above are increased 7-fold in the cervical area, and 5- to 2.3-fold in the thoracic and lumbar areas. This illustrates the positive effect of powerfully developed spinal muscles and of stable ligaments on the load-bearing capacity of a normally shaped spinal column, because **it reduces the load pressure on the vertebrae and the intervertebral discs by a factor of 5–6!**

After the straightening of the trunk (in the 3rd year of life), the intervertebral disc (discus intervertebralis) loses its blood vessels and neurons and can tolerate this increased mechanical pressure only because

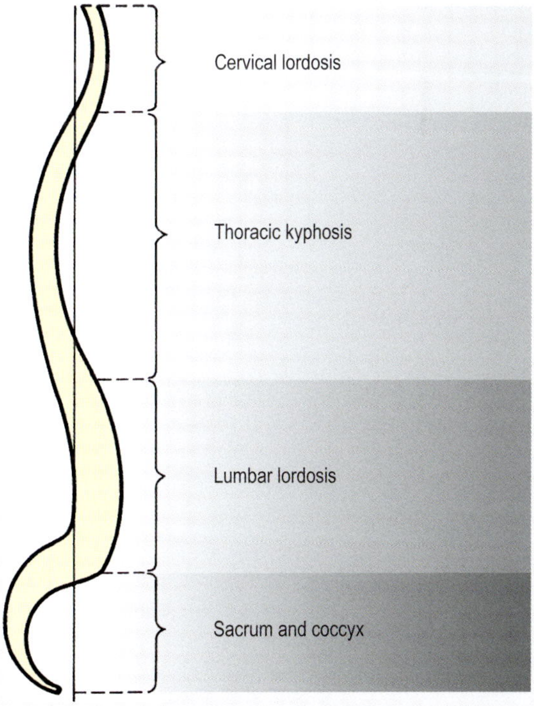

Fig. 18 The physiological curvatures of the spinal column.

of its special microstructure. This consists (fig. 19) of a fibro-cartilaginous ring (anulus fibrosus), surrounding a gelatinous core (nucleus pulposus). The latter is characterized by high water content and by flexibility. Together they determine its hydrostatic effectiveness ("water-cushion-function"), which is maintained by the tonicity of the fibro-cartilaginous ring and by the tone of the muscles of the spinal column. The intervertebral disc and the adjacent vertebral bodies are connected by a **hyaline cartilage plate**. This plate demarcates the vertebral body from above and below, and acts as a semipermeable membrane for the **diffusion of liquids** into the intervertebral disc (and vice versa). In this way the **nutrition of the intervertebral disc** is guaranteed, when it is subjected to a constant change of axial strain and relief of that strain.

With age and lack of mobility the gelatinous core undergoes biochemical changes: increase of nitrogen content, increased loss of water-binding hyaluronic acid, which lead to a decrease in the internal pressure of the intervertebral disc. As a consequence it loses its jelly-like quality and ability

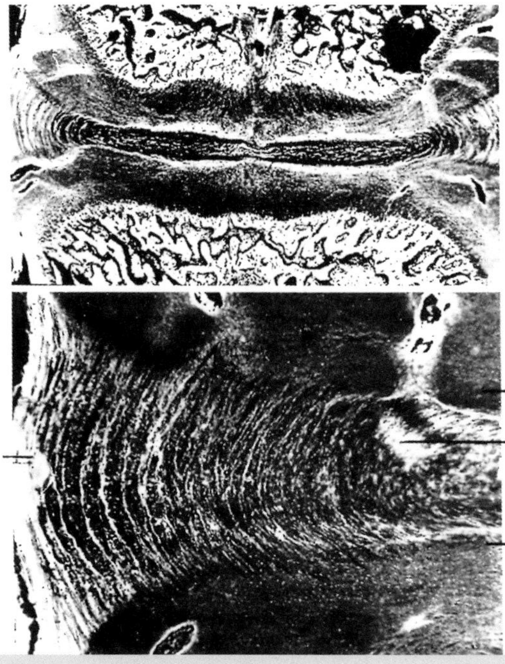

Fig. 19 A general view of the intervertebral disc (a) and enlarged details (b).

1 = hyaline cartilage, semi-permeable plate
2 = fibro-cartilage lamellae (anulus fibrosus)
3 = gelatinous core (nucleus pulposus)

to distribute the axial load evenly over the intervertebral disc. This leads to a **decrease in mechanical weight-bearing capacity.**

The relatively "soft" cushioning effect is caused by the double S-shape of the spinal column in the median and sagittal plane, on which the position of the pelvis has a significant influence (lumbar spinal column and sacral bone form an angle of 143°). This **leads to less strain** on the intervertebral discs and intervertebral joints.

Because of the approximately equal size of two intervertebral articular bodies as well as of the flattened joint surfaces, which are surrounded by tight articular capsules with short reinforcing ligaments, only restricted movement is possible against each other for the individual joint connections of the spinal column (with the exception of the atlanto-occipital and atlanto-axial joints). Only the **totality** of these partial movements and the elasticity of the total of 23 fibrocartilaginous intervertebral discs result in a relatively high degree of **all-round mobility of the central axial skeleton**, which can often vary enormously between the different individual sections.

The following **main directions of movements of the spinal column** (and as a consequence of the trunk) can be distinguished:

- a forward and backward flexion around the transversal axis (= anteversion and retroversion), which is particularly pronounced in the cervical and lumbar spinal column,
- a lateral inclination around the sagittal axis (= lateroflexion), which is perfectly feasible in the area of the cervical and thoracic spinal column, and
- a torsion around the vertical axis (= rotation), which is particularly well developed and can reach 80–90° in the cervical and thoracic part of the axial skeleton – almost invariably in connection with a slight lateral inclination of the head or the trunk to the same side.

The structure of the spinal column outlined above makes it possible to transfer **the entire weight of the upper half of the body on to the pelvic girdle.** This is facilitated by the fact that the sacral bone (os sacrum) is part of the structure of the spinal column. Because of these anatomical preconditions, according to which the central axial skeleton must accomodate all the movements of the pelvis in the hip joints in relation to the lower extremities, it is in a **constantly unstable equilibrium**. This is maintained by the short and the long dorsal muscles (m. erector spinae), located in the furrows to the right and left of the spinous-process line, as well as by the abdominal muscles, the iliopsoas and the scaleni, all of which are on the anterior surface of the trunk. In this way the whole spinal column is subjected to the interplay of the anterior and posterior muscle masses, which make **falling forwards or backwards** practically impossible.

Mollier (1938) and Benninghoff (1954) have compared the protection of the upright posture by the muscle strands with the rigging of the mast of a ship, which is similar to the "tension-rod" principle used in scaffolding. In the illustration (fig. 20) the spreaders of the mast correspond to the transversal processes of the axial skeleton, which are connected with one another by short muscles. The muscular rigging also runs diagonally from the ends of the spreaders to the mast, and occasionally leaves out some segments. Apart from these short muscle strands, to which the delicate, paired muscles which connect the spinous processes in the cervical and lumbar spine also belong, the illustration of the

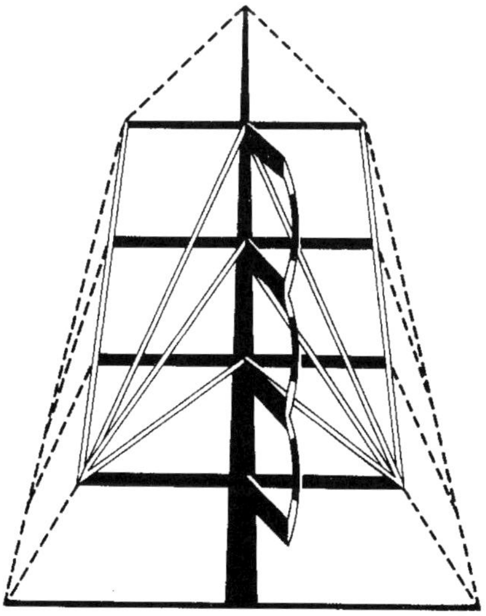

Fig. 20 Illustration of the structure of the deep dorsal muscles superimposed on the drawing of the mast of a ship. Base: pelvis = deck of the ship, horizontal lines = transversal spinous processes (guy), connecting lines = muscle strands (tension ropes).

mast of the ship also shows long, "guys" (muscles), which run from the deck of the ship – the pelvic girdle – to the spreaders.

Fig. 20 shows the marvellous way in which the individual vertebrae and their bony processes are anchored by the muscles to one another and all of them to the pelvic girdle and the ribs. If we take into consideration that all these muscle strands – even when the body is completely at rest – are in a state of constant tension (tone), we can easily see that with a movement of the trunk which seems so simple and which involves the shortening of at least some muscle strands, other muscles must be relaxed, and others must be extended. This leads to a **continuous readjustment of the whole system** to bring the central axial skeleton, by actively adjustable "rigging", constantly into its new position and to secure it at the same time. That means: **the trunk and the spinal column,** which are continuously involved in the movements and the loads put on the whole body, are **a functional unity,** in which the individual constituents can only be understood and assessed in the context of the arrangement and function of the whole.

Short and long muscles of the spinal column

The strong muscles of the spinal column **(erector spinae)** are subdivided into two large groups, one of which is confined to the spinal column, and the other is located laterally to it.

- The **deep medial muscle strand** is composed of powerful short- to medium-length muscle groups, which connect the spinous and transverse processes. These are in particular
  - the interspinal muscles (interspinales),
  - the intertransversal muscles (intertransversarii),
  - the rotator muscles (rotatores),
  - the fan-shapes muscles (multifidi) and
  - the semispinalis muscle (semispinalis).

  These muscles have **dynamic** functions:
  - when bilaterally contracted, extension and stabilization of the spinal column,
  - when unilaterally contracted, lateral inclination and rotation of the spinal column.

  They also perform **static** functions such as a

gentle deceleration of movements, at the right moment, before their final position is reached.

- The **superficial lateral muscle group,** the sacrospinalis, which constitutes the main body of the spinal muscles, consists of two muscles, which become progressively narrower when they extend cranially from the lumbar part of the axial skeleton,
  - the more medially situated long muscles of the back **(longissimus)** and
  - the laterally situated muscles connecting the ilium with the ribs **(iliocostalis).**

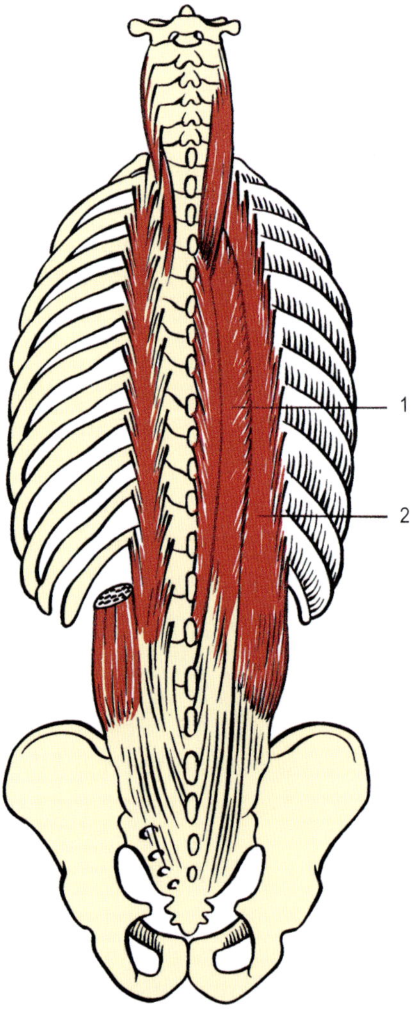

1 long dorsal muscle (longissimus)
2 iliac rib muscle (iliocostalis)

Fig. 21 The lateral strand of the spinal muscles.

The **long dorsal muscle** (longissimus, fig. 21) originates with strong muscle strands from the sacral bone (sacrum) and the iliac crest (crista iliaca), and is attached to the transversal processes of the lower thoracic vertebrae and lower ribs. Here it acquires new (accessory) points of origin, which extend the muscle to the lower cervical spinal column. It acquires further points of origin on the transversal processes of the upper thoracic and lower cervical segments and continues on to the mastoid process of the temporal bone (processus mastoideus). As a consequence the long muscle consists of 3–4 muscle sections which overlap like tiles on a roof.

The **iliocostalis** (fig. 21) which has been largely displaced from the spinal column, originates mainly from the iliac crest and has its first points of attachment to the lower ribs. Here it acquires new points of origin and continues to the 6 upper ribs. The iliocostalis terminates after this middle section with its muscle strands attached to the transversal processes of the 4th–6th cervical vertebrae.

The **function of both muscles,** when contracted bilaterally, is to extend the central axial skeleton powerfully, and, when contracted unilaterally, to incline it to the same side.

The short and long muscle fibres of the inner and outer strand of the erector spinae are united by a layer of dense connective tissue which is particularly well developed in the lumbar region, the diamond-shaped **fascia thoracolumbalis,** bundled together to form a single structure and connected to the spinal column (fig. 22 and 23). It plays an important part in **regulating and stabilizing the posture of the body,** because it serves as a point of origin, with its superficial layer, for the broad dorsal muscle – the latissimus dorsi, and the serratus posterior inferior – and with its deep inner layer for the transversus abdominis and obliquus abdominis internus.

The cumulative effect of the muscles of the spinal column and the effect of gravity

In order to get an overview of the cumulative effect of the muscles of the spinal column, it is important to take into consideration the influence of gravity.

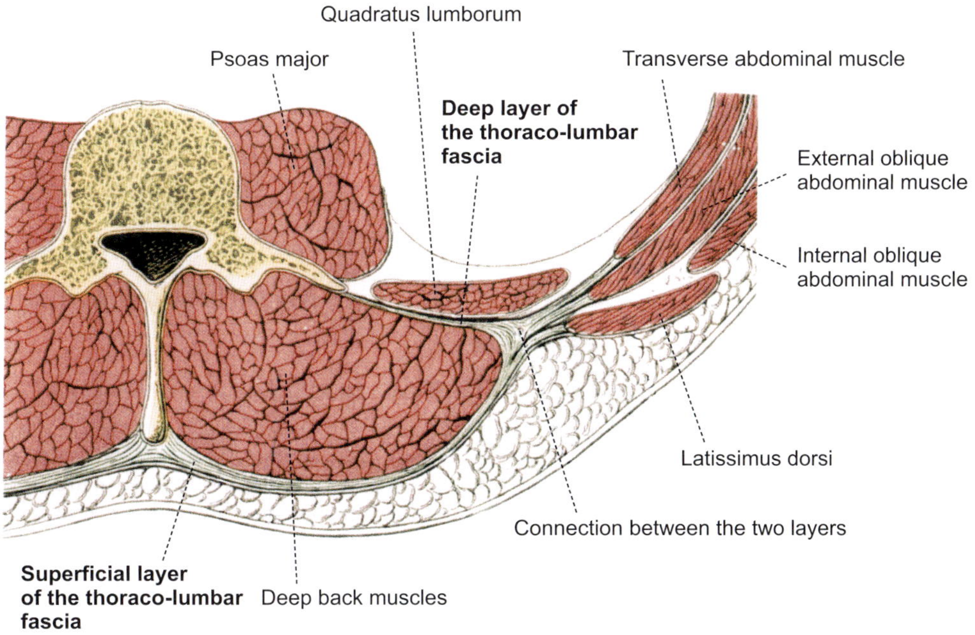

Fig. 22 Cross-section through the torso at the level of the lower thoracic and lumbar region, which shows the thoraco-lumbar fascia with the connection between its superficial and deep layers, and the structural links with the transversus abdominis and obliquus internus adominis and the latissimus dorsi.

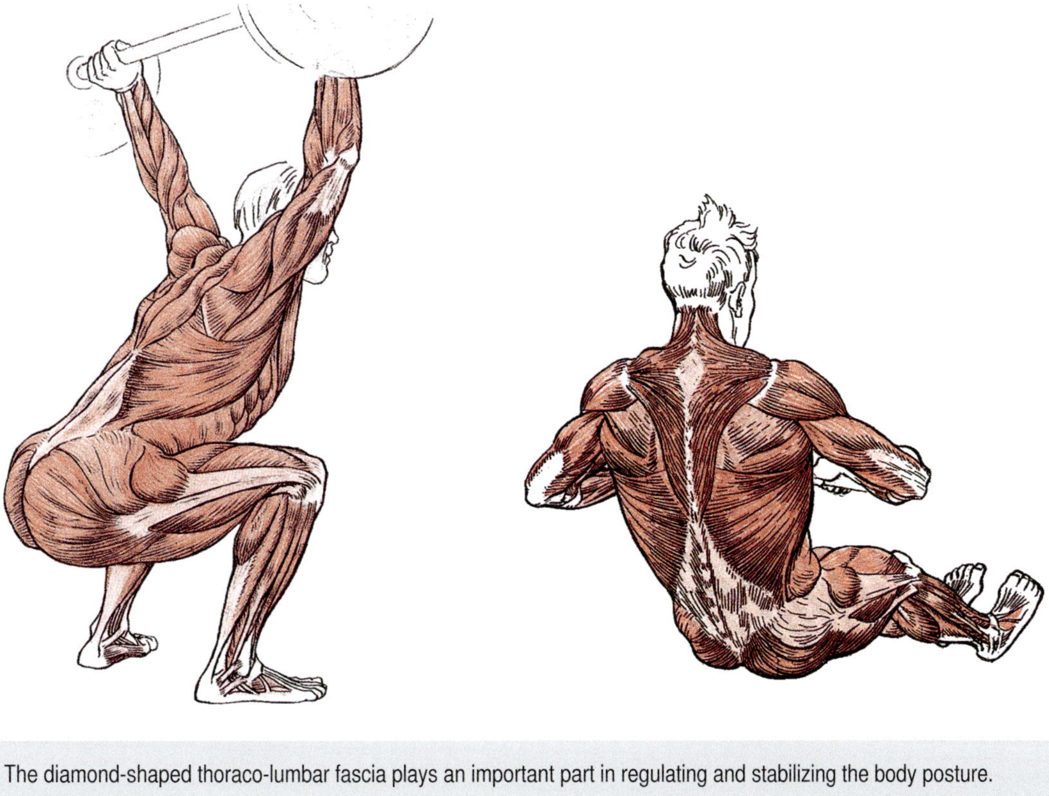

Fig. 23 The diamond-shaped thoraco-lumbar fascia plays an important part in regulating and stabilizing the body posture.

Gravity sometimes operates against the intended movement and sometimes with it. When the trunk is bent forward (ventral flexion), its weight tends to bend it even further forward. The deep dorsal muscles, which consist mainly of short fibres with a large physiological cross-section, and the powerful large gluteal muscle (gluteus maximus), are, in this position, under considerably increased tension. This determines the extent to which the upper body can be held in a position of forward inclination, or the extent to which the trunk can be bent down even further when the tension diminishes. The muscle masses bulging on both sides of the lumbar spinal column illustrate this "battle" of the muscles mentioned above against the weight of the body when the trunk is inclined forward.

The forward inclination of the trunk has three stages:

- in the first stage, the thorax and the shoulder girdle, including the upper extremities, are pulled down or forward by the strength of the **straight and oblique abdominal muscles** (fig. 24),
- secondly – and this particularly applies to the lumbar spinal column and the pelvis – this section of the **iliopsoas** is contracted (fig. 25), and,
- thirdly, the short and long strands of the **spinal muscles** (erector spinae, fig. 26) with the large **gluteal muscles** (fig. 25) regulate the forward flexion of the trunk by means of their very variable tension, although in the anatomical literature they are described exclusively as dorsal extensor muscles!

The strongest muscle masses causing this movement are situated in the region of the lumbar and cervical spinal column (fig. 26), which, by the strength of their contraction, bring about the lordotic curvature of these sections (see above).

The same applies to the **backward extension and lateral flexion of the trunk.** Once the contraction of the muscles initiates the movement, it is continued by the weight of the upper body. The resistance of the following muscles diminishes to work against gravity by regulating these movements and preventing extreme movements:

- in the case of over-extension the anterior musculature of the body (see fig. 28),
- in the case of lateral inclination of the trunk the muscles of the convex part of the body (fig. 27).

This interrelationship between muscle tension on the one hand, and gravity on the other, illustrates once again that every movement of the body is never an isolated event, but is always an indication of the performance of the body as a whole.

It is the muscles of the trunk which are particularly involved in the movement of the whole body. Their action precedes the action of the upper extremities in dynamic movements (for example throwing a javelin) and this can be regarded as an initial movement.

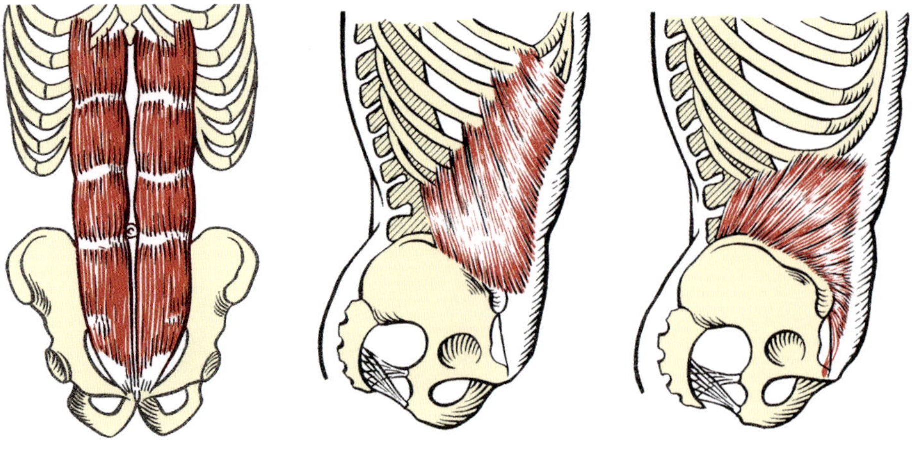

Fig. 24 Rectus abdominis muscle (left), external (middle) and internal (right) oblique muscles.

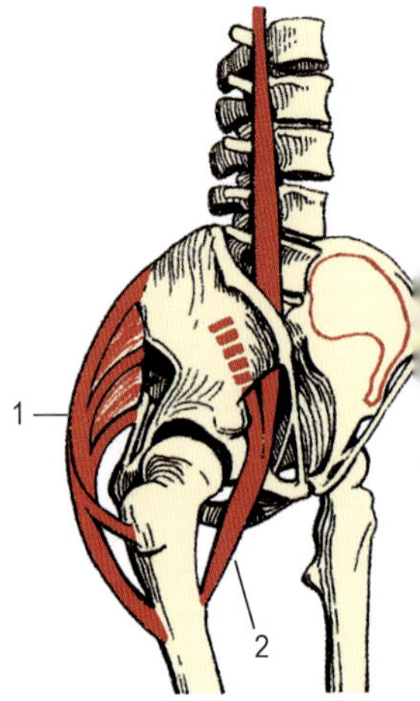

Fig. 25 Gluteus maximus (1) an
psoas (2).

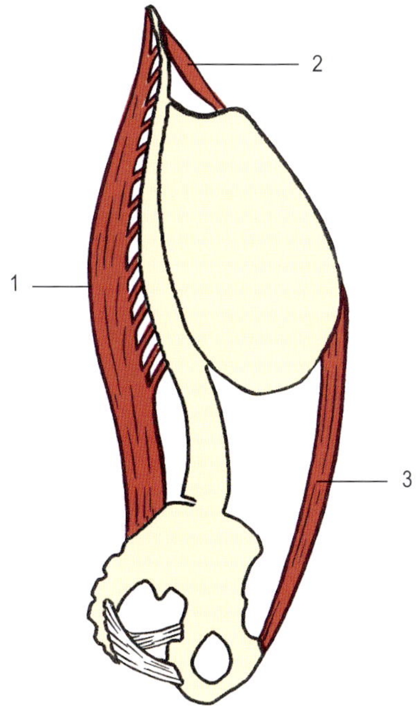

1 erector spinae muscles
2 cervical muscles (scaleni and sternocleidomastoid)
3 rectus abdominis

Fig. 26 Rectus abdominis (for the flexion) and erector spinae (for the extension) of the spinal column in the forward and backward inclination of the trunk.

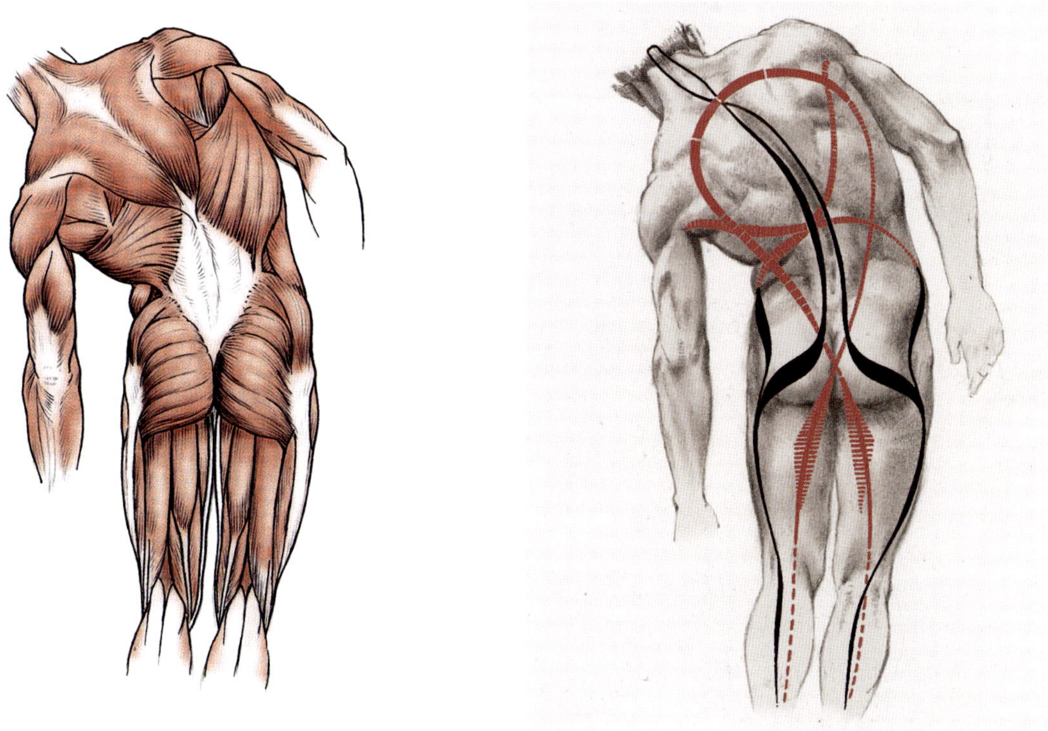

Fig. 27 In lateral inclination of the body the muscles of the convex side work against gravity.

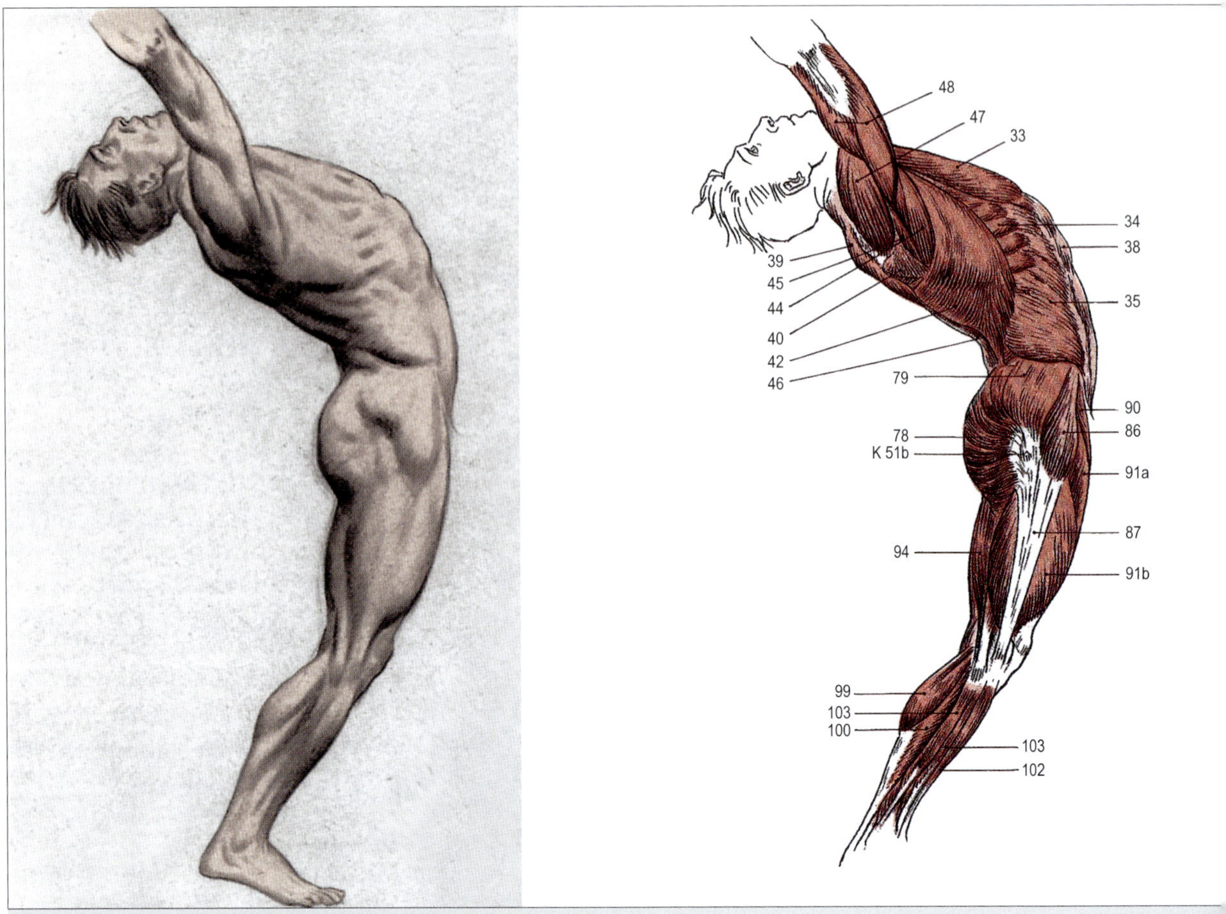

Fig. 28 Overextension of the body backwards.

2.2 Extensor slings in whole-body movements

Overextension of the body backwards

As demonstrated in the basic movement of the extensor sling over the whole of the body during backwards flexion of the trunk (fig. 28) and in one phase of the sequence of movements of a slender long-distance runner (fig. 29), the extensor sling marked in the diagram does not terminate at the iliac crest, as opposed to the movements shown in fig. 29, but continues into the long and short deep dorsal muscles (erector spinae). The course of the sling of the antagonists continues in the same way on the anterior side of the trunk into the area of the rectus abdominis. Fig. 28 shows that the lower leg is significantly pushed forward by the tibialis anterior and the pelvis by the traction effect of the biceps femoris and the semitendinosus at the tuber of the ischium, in order to maintain the balance of the over-stretched trunk, and so of the whole body. Which muscles have to be activated to fixate the body in its current position or to bring it back to its original position?

Fig. 28 shows the very powerful contraction of the deep dorsal muscles (erector spinae) which initiates the backwards flexion of the trunk, which will then be continued immediately afterwards by the weight of the trunk. At the same time as the over-extension of the central axial skeleton – this illustrates what

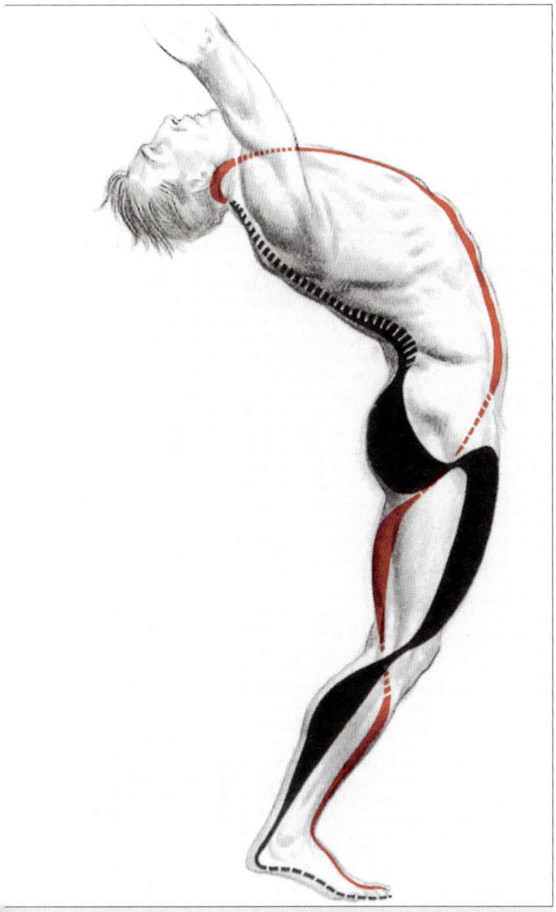

Muscles Fig. 28

33	Pectoralis major	**79**	Gluteus medius
34	Serratus anterior	**86**	Tensor fasciae latae
35	Obliquus externus abdominis	**87**	Tractus iliotibialis
		90	Sartorius
38	Rectus abdominis	**91a**	Rectus femoris
39	Trapezius	**91b**	Vastus lateralis
40	Supra- et infraspinatus	**94**	Biceps femoris
42	Latissimus dorsi	**99**	Gastrocnemius
44	Teres major	**100**	Soleus
45	Teres minor	**102**	Tibialis anterior
46	Erector spinae	**103**	Extensor digitorum longus
47	Deltoideus		
48	Triceps brachii		
78	Gluteus maximus	**K51b**	Trochanter major

we have already learnt, which is that every change in a single element leads as a consequence to an adjustment of the whole – there is a flattening and increasing extension of the abdominal and thoracic muscles. As soon as the backward flexion of the trunk, by the long and short dorsal muscles, has reached a point at which only the weight of the body has an effect, then the **antagonists must increase their tension:**

- the rectus abdominis, supported by the obliquus abdominis externus and internus muscles and
- the pectoralis major on both sides of the body.

They must increase their extension to such an extent that the upper body either remains in the over-flexed backward position (and is thus prevented from falling) or can return to its normal starting position by means of contraction. The muscles mentioned above are supported in this by the scaleni and the sternocleidomastoid. The more the work of the deep dorsal muscles done in extending and over-extending is reduced by the increasing effect of gravity, the greater the tension of the abdominal and thoracic muscles must be increased to **maintain the necessary muscular balance.**

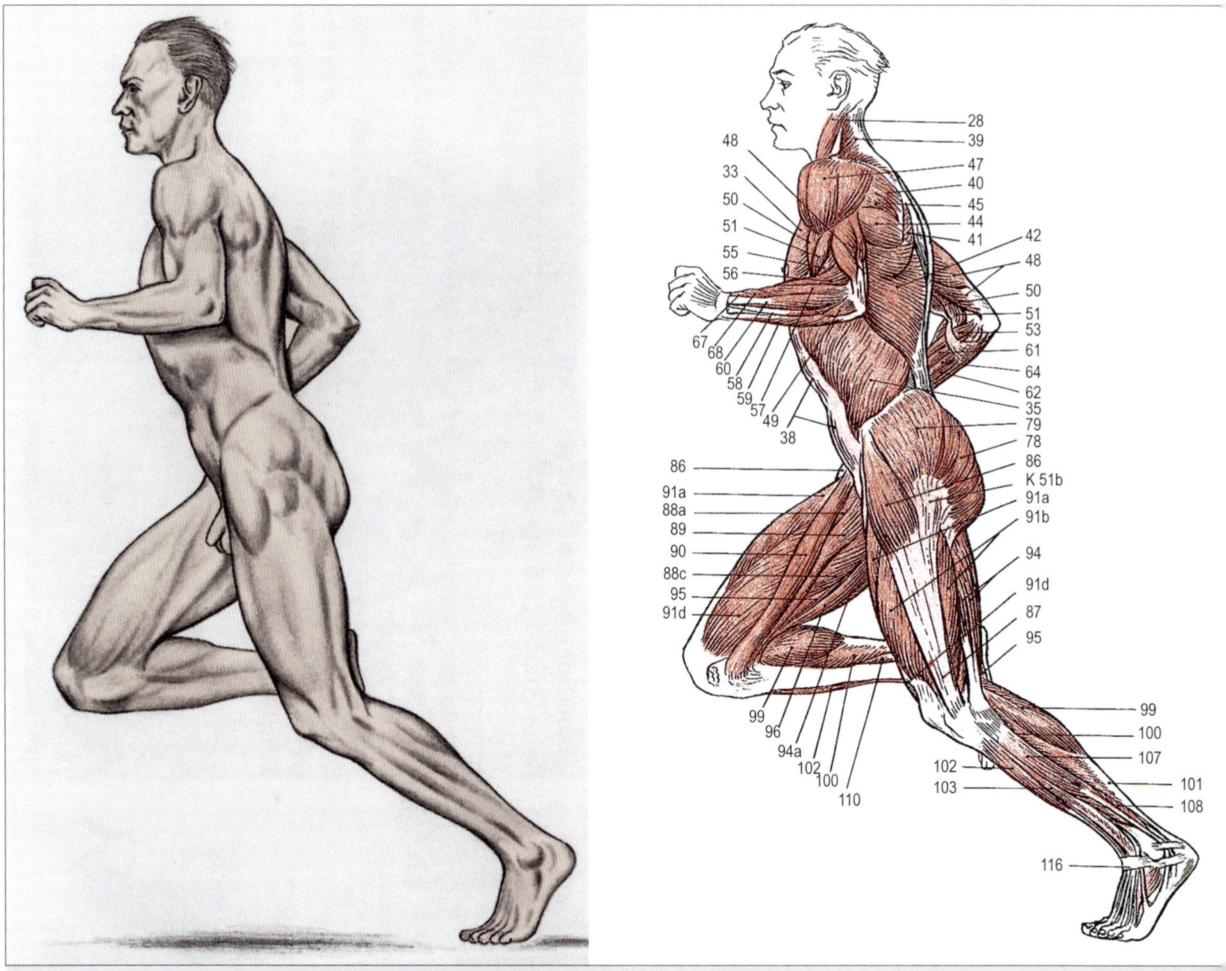

Fig. 29 Extensor sling over the whole of the body in a long-distance runner.

Long- and middle-distance runners

If we follow the extensor sling in the long- and middle-distance runner (fig. 29 and 30), we can identify, in the pushing off and supporting phase, three sections of the sling which run from the heel to the iliac crest. It should also be mentioned that the posterior-muscle strands of the adductor magnus – as opposed to the other adductors of the thigh – take part in the extension process. The function of the gluteus maximus is taken over, not only by the latissimus dorsi, but also by the erector spinae and the multifidi via the fascia thoracolumbalis (fig. 22, 23).

The architecture of the slings in the long-distance runner (fig. 29), who as a rule is a "heel runner", who touches down with the outer edge of the foot and rolls it inwardly with a pronation movement, also illustrates the load put on the muscles of the calf and the foot: the **seven plantar flexors** (gastrocnemius, soleus, flexor hallucis longus, fibularis longus et brevis, tibialis posterior and flexor digitorum longus).

They develop four times as much power as the **three dorsal extensors** (tibialis anterior, extensor digitorum longus, extensor hallucis longus) – which are also very important for standing since they work against the centre of gravity of the body – which are used especially by short- and middle-distance runners who are "ball-of-the-foot runners". The muscular balance and the transversal arch of the foot are secured by the functional unity of the fib-

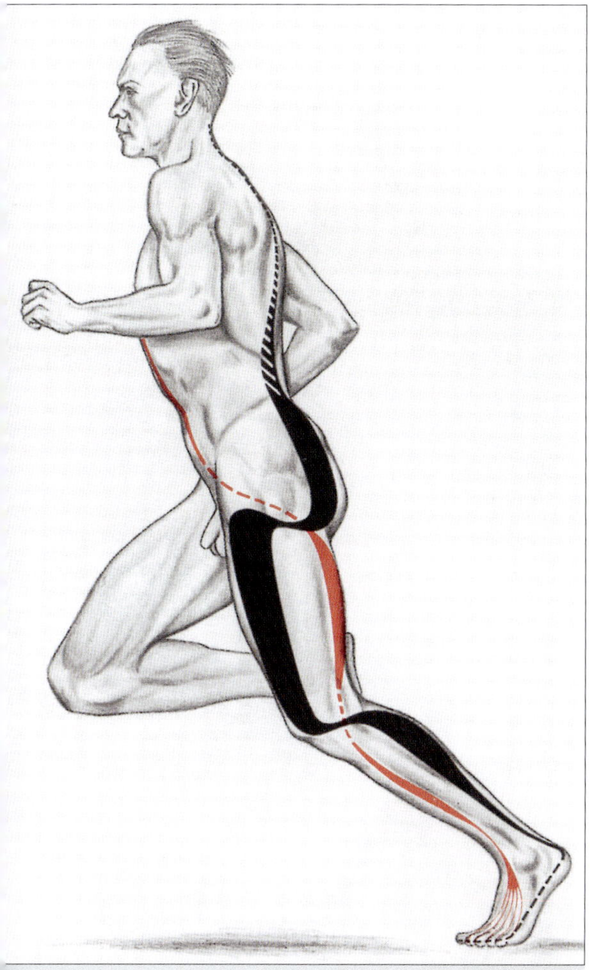

Muscles Fig. 29

28 Sternocleidomastoideus
33 Pectoralis major
35 Obliquus externus abdominis
38 Rectus abdominis
39 Trapezius
40 Supra- et infraspinatus
41 Rhomboideus major
42 Latissimus dorsi
44 Teres major
45 Teres minor
47 Deltoideus
48 Triceps brachii
49 Anconeus
50 Biceps brachii
51 Brachialis
53 Pronator teres
55 Brachioradialis
56 Extensor carpi radialis longus
57 Extensor carpi radialis brevis
58 Extensor carpi ulnaris
59 Flexor carpi ulnaris
60 Extensor digitorum
61 Brachioradialis
62 Flexor digitorum superficialis
64 Palmaris longus
67 Extensor pollicis brevis
68 Abductor pollicis longus
78 Gluteus maximus
79 Gluteus medius
86 Tensor fasciae latae
87 Tractus iliotibialis
88a Adductor longus
88c Adductor magnus
89 Gracilis
90 Sartorius
91a Rectus femoris
91b Vastus lateralis
91d Vastus intermedius
94 Biceps femoris
94a Biceps femoris, caput longum
95 Semimembranosus
96 Semitendinosus
99 Gastrocnemius
100 Soleus
101 Tendo calcaneus
102 Tibialis anterior
103 Extensor digitorum longus
107 Fibularis longus
108 Fibularis brevis
110 Flexor digitorum longus
116 Retinaculum musculorum extensorum superius

K51b Trochanter major

ularis longus and the tibialis anterior, which form a tendinous and muscular "stirrup".

The "brake sling" is composed of the muscles of the anterior lower leg and the posterior thigh, which continues on, via the main part of the adductors of the thigh, to the symphysis, and from there to the rectus abdominis.

This combination of muscle groups is then continued

- in the abdominal fascial part of the pectoralis major and
- via the interposed sternum to the sternocleidomastoideus and the scaleni muscles (see above).

After demonstrating these basic movements we will show some examples of extensor slings over the whole of the body (with their corresponding antagonists).

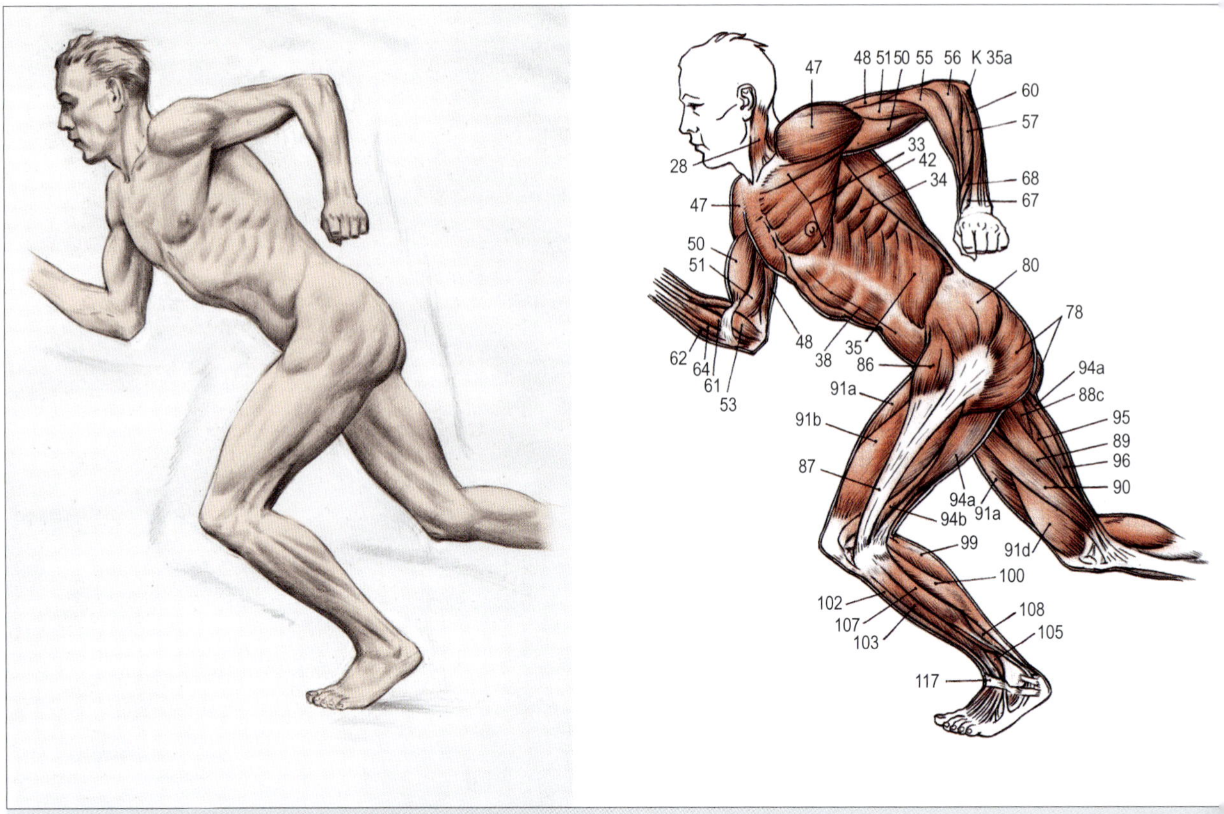

Fig. 30 Extensor sling over the whole of the body in a middle-distance runner.

Anthropometric characteristics are important preconditions for high performance in many sport disciplines. This also applies to the different kinds of long-distance running (tables 1–3).

Table 1: Average body height (m) of Olympic middle-distance runners.

	Men		Women	
	all	6 finalists	all	6 finalists
400 m	1.79	1.82	1.68	1.68
800 m	1.78	1.79	1.67	1.68
1.500 m	1.77	1.77	1.66	1.68

Table 2: Average body weight (kg) of Olympic middle-distance runners.

	Men		Women	
	all	6 finalists	all	6 finalists
400 m	75.2	73.2	56.2	56.8
800 m	72.2	69.4	57.2	56.6
1.500 m	68.0	68.0	55.2	54.4

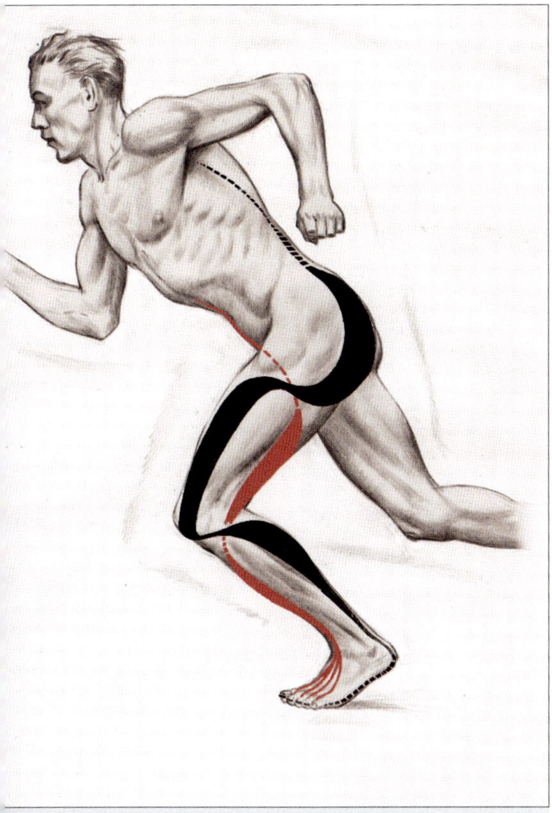

Muscles Fig. 30

28 Sternocleidomastoideus
33 Pectoralis major
34 Serratus anterior
35 Obliquus externus abdominis
38 Rectus abdominis
42 Latissimus dorsi
47 Deltoideus
48 Triceps brachii
48a Caput laterale tricipitis brachii
50 Biceps brachii
51 Brachialis
53 Pronator teres
55 Brachioradialis
56 Extensor carpi radialis longus
57 Extensor carpi radialis brevis
60 Extensor digitorum
61 Flexor carpi radialis
62 Flexor digitorum superficialis
64 Palmaris longus
67 Extensor pollicis brevis
68 Abductor pollicis longus
78 Gluteus maximus
80 Gluteus minimus
86 Tensor fasciae latae
87 Tractus iliotibialis
88c Adductor magnus
89 Gracilis
90 Sartorius
91a Rectus femoris
91b Vastus lateralis
94a Biceps femoris, caput longum
94b Biceps femoris, caput breve
95 Semimembranosus
96 Semitendinosus
99 Gastrocnemius
100 *Soleus*
102 Tibialis anterior
103 Extensor digitorum longus
105 Fibularis tertius
107 Fibularis longus
108 Fibularis brevis
110 Flexor digitorum longus
117 Retinaculum musculorum extensorum superius

K35a Olecranon

Table 3: Anthropometrical and muscle-cellular differences between middle-distance runners of both sexes.

	Women	Men
Age (years)	20	20
Body height (m)	1.69	1.80
Body mass (kg)	57.0	67.0
$V0_2$ max (ml/kg x min)	69.0	72.0
Muscle fibre type (%)		
Slow twitch	68	73
Fast twitch	32	27
Muscles fibre area (µm²)	5440	7040

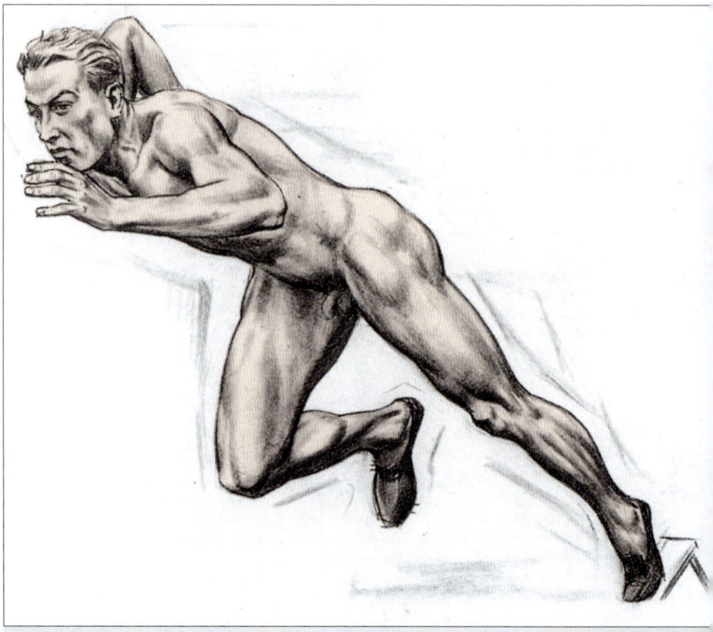

Fig. 31 Whole-body extensor sling in a sprinter at the start of the 100 meters.

Sprinter (at the start of the 100 meters)

There is an interesting sequence of movements at the start of the 100 meters in track-and-field athletics (fig. 31). The sprinter starts from a crouched position with the trunk bent forward (the centre of gravity of the body of the sprinter is in the thoracic region) with a pronounced flexion of the hip, knee and upper-ankle joints. The angle of the knee joint of a sprinter in the starting phase is 70–100° for the front leg and 100–120° for the back leg.

In this position – as also seen in the initial jump of the swimmer who has a knee-joint angle of 150–170° (fig. 32) – there is a **strong pre-extension** of the extensors and optimization of the appropriate angles, which are a condition **for strong and fast contraction.**

As soon as the starting signal has been given the front leg (the left leg in the illustration) is extended and at the same time the back leg (the right leg) is pressed hard against the ground and then pulled forward with lightning speed, and this increases the thrust even more which has been achieved by the explosive extension of the front leg. This exact moment in the movement is shown in the illustration (fig. 31). The explosive pushing-off from the starting block by the hip, knee and ankle extensors united in a whole-body extensor sling comes about with a power of 1100–1250 N in the sprinter and, after only a few paces, reaches 92–95 % of the top speed during the starting and acceleration phase.

It is a well-know fact that the **high performance of the world's best sprinters** (100 m in 9.58 sec!) is achieved by a pronounced and long-lasting accelerative capability, by high maximum speed as well as lack of rigidity (in the phase of maximum speed as a pre-condition of fighting for the best position in the final straight) and by a perfectly honed technique (crouch start, sprint technique for reaching the finishing line).

The importance of a well-developed accelerative and lightning-speed capability which is a condition of achieving top speed, makes it necessary to

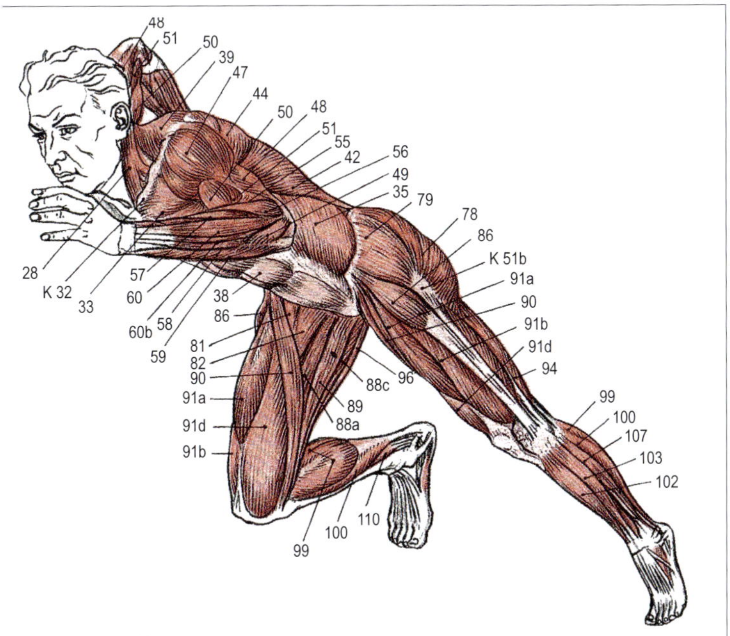

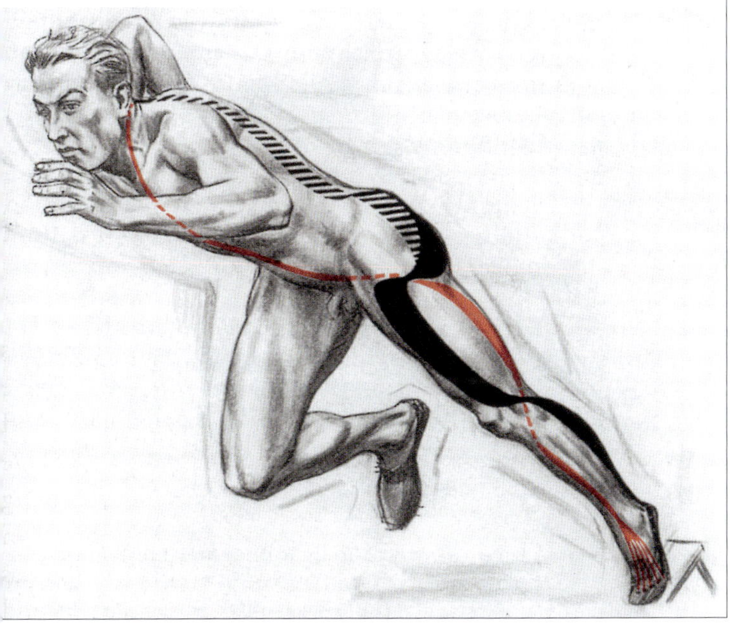

Muscles Fig. 31

28 Sternocleidomastoideus
33 Pectoralis major
35 Obliquus externus abdominis
38 Rectus abdominis
39 Trapezius
42 Latissimus dorsi
44 Teres major
47 Deltoideus
48 Triceps brachii
49 Anconeus
50 Biceps brachii
51 Brachialis
55 Brachioradialis
56 Extensor carpi radialis longus
57 Extensor carpi radialis brevis
58 Extensor carpi ulnaris
59 Flexor carpi ulnaris
60 Extensor digitorum
60b Abductor digiti minimi
78 Gluteus maximus
79 Gluteus medius
81 Iliopsoas
82 Pectineus
86 Tensor fasciae latae
88a Adductor longus
88c Adductor magnus
89 Gracilis
90 Sartorius
91a Rectus femoris
91b Vastus lateralis
91d Vastus intermedius
94 Biceps femoris
96 Semitendinosus
99 Gastrocnemius
100 Soleus
102 Tibialis anterior
103 Extensor digitorum longus
107 Fibularis longus
110 Flexor digitorum longus

K32 Clavicula
K51b Trochanter major

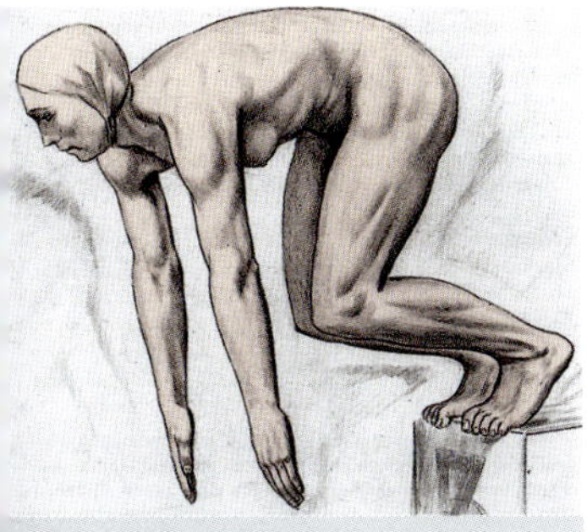

Fig. 32 Initial jump of the swimmer.

deploy training resources to develop sprint-power endurance, maximum power and lightning power specific to the type of sport. This applies especially to the strength training of the trunk and arms, and to jumping and stretching exercises, as a basis for the athlete's all-round muscle training. The periods of the individual strength training overlap with further training using the previous training methods at the same level of performance. Maximum strength is dependent on a large muscle-fibre cross-section, on the pre-dominance of "fast" muscle fibres (fast-twitch fibres) and on the fast voluntary synchronization of multiple muscle fibres.

This strength potential which determines sprinting performance is shown in the naturalistic illustration of the starting sprinter (fig. 31). The muscles responsible for the extension of the lower extremity bulge below the surface of the body in the form of more or less clearly developed round or longish protrusions, which can be identified with the knowledge we have acquired so far.

The following structures are particularly noticeable:

- the pronounced heads of the gastrocnemius and
- the soleus bulging from under this muscle
- with their shared tendinous component of the powerful achilles tendon, which is particularly noticeable against its surrounding tissue, which contains very little fat
- the powerful muscle-mass of the quadriceps
- the pronounced lateral surface of the gluteus maximus
- the tensor fasciae latae with the Maissiat band (tractus iliotibialis) and
- the deep short and long dorsal muscles (erector spinae).

If we look at the naturalistic drawing (fig. 31) it becomes clear that the accompanying **movements of the arms alternate with the movements of the legs.** These arm movements pull up the body of the runner starting from a low crouching position during which – as one can see with the right arm – can even lead to backward movements. We have the impression that both arms are performing movements as if they were pushing away some resistance in the air.

The contribution of the upper extremities to the forward movement of the body decreases with the length of the running distance, without completely disappearing. This is because in the process of running as well as the stabilization of the equilibrium of the body during the "flight phase" of the long- and middle-distance runner (fig. 33) the contribution of the upper extremities cannot be discounted completely.

The course of the extensor and "brake" slings in the runner at the start is basically the same as shown in the basic movement (fig. 33) – however with very variable application of strength. The extensor muscles try to bring the over-inclined body into an upright position against the force of gravity, and the centre of gravity of the body back to the pelvis.

Muscles Fig. 33

28 Sternocleidomastoideus
33 Pectoralis major
34 Serratus anterior
35 Obliquus externus abdominis
38 Rectus abdominis
39 Trapezius
40 Supra- et infraspinatus
41 Rhomboideus major
42 Latissimus dorsi
44 Teres major
45 Teres minor
47 Deltoideus
48 Triceps brachii
48a Caput laterale m. tricipitis brachii
49 Anconeus
50 Biceps brachii
51 Brachialis
53 Pronator teres
55 Brachioradialis
56 Extensor carpi radialis longus
57 Extensor carpi radialis brevis
58 Extensor carpi ulnaris
59 Flexor carpi ulnaris
60 Extensor digitorum
60b Abductor digiti minimi
61 Brachioradialis
62 Flexor digitorum superficialis
64 Palmaris longus
67 Extensor pollicis brevis
68 Abductor pollicis longus
78 Gluteus maximus
79 Gluteus medius
80 Gluteus minimus
81 Iliopsoas
82 Pectineus
86 Tensor fasciae latae
87 Tractus iliotibialis
88a Adductor longus
88c Adductor magnus
89 Gracilis
90 Sartorius
91a Rectus femoris
91b Vastus lateralis
91c Vastus medialis
91d Vastus intermedius
94 Biceps femoris
94a Biceps femoris, caput longum
94b Biceps femoris, caput breve abdominis
95 Semimembranosus
96 Semitendinosus
99 Gastrocnemius
100 Soleus
101 Tendo calcaneus
102 Tibialis anterior
103 Extensor digitorum longus
104 Extensor digitorum brevis
105 Fibularis tertius
107 Fibularis longus
108 Fibularis brevis
110 Flexor digitorum longus
116/117 Retinaculum musculorum extensorum superior

K32 Clavicula
K35a Olecranon
K46 Spina iliaca anterior superior
K51b Trochanter major
K53 Patella

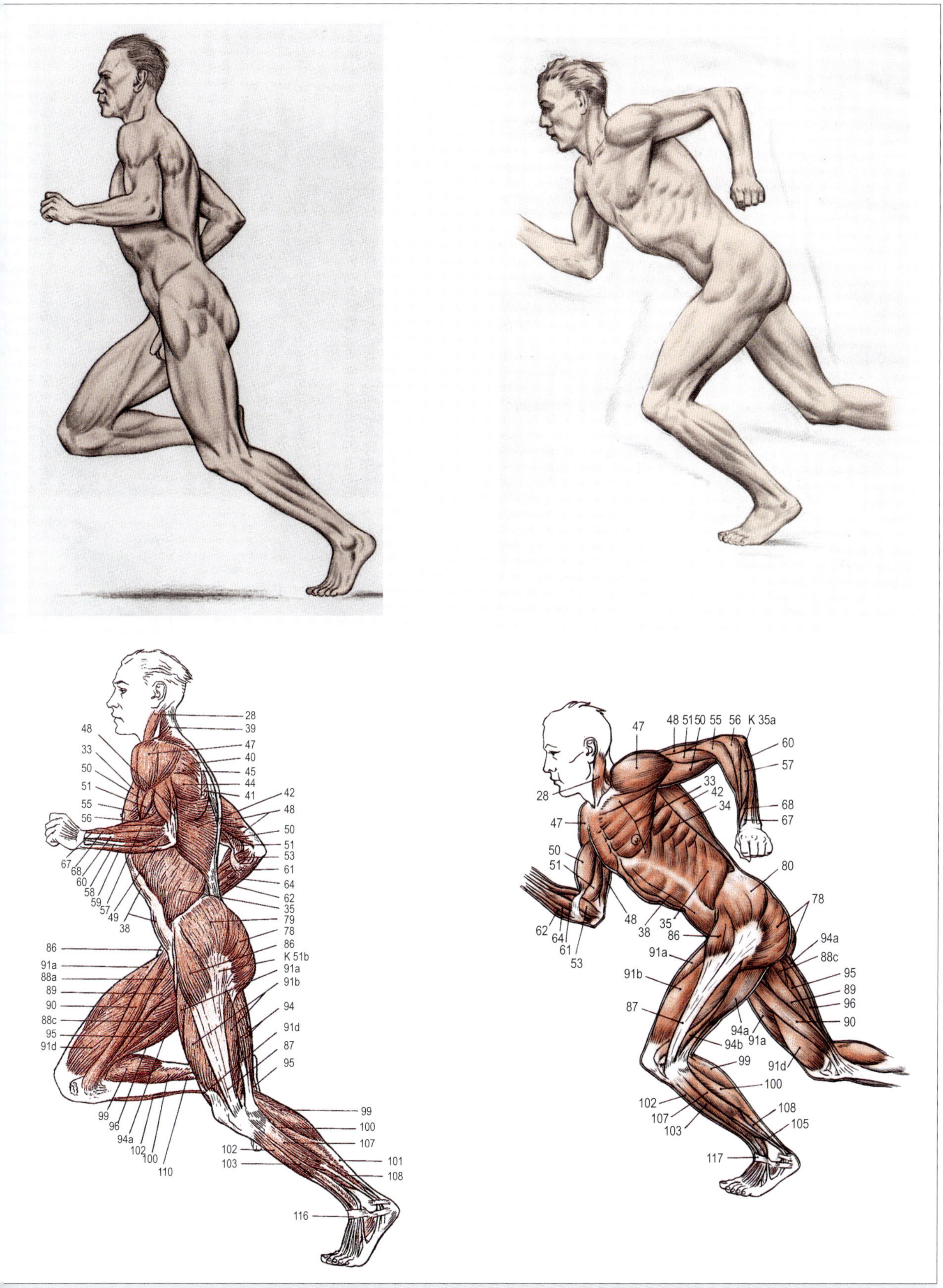

Fig. 33 The long- and middle-distance runners demonstrate yet again the whole-body movement and, in particularl, the action of the powerful muscles of the lower extremity.

Javelin thrower

Before we discuss the next illustration, the javelin thrower (fig. 34) some introductory remarks are necessary. It is well-known that the technique of throwing the javelin has four phases – the starting phase, the running-up phase (with a loose, cyclic acceleration and an acyclic five-step rhythm), the throwing phase and the braking phase. The illustration shows the moment when there is a marked hyperextension of the lumbar spine as well as a maximal arching of the body up to the start of the slingshot of the lower part of the throwing arm. This imposing **arching of the body,** which at any moment will be released with a whipping-flinging forward and upward movement of the arm, is very similar to the explosive release of a coiled spring. This comparison also applies to the drawing and releasing of a bow.

In the naturalistic drawing (fig. 34) the foot of the maximally extended left leg reached its final position before the throw. At the same time there is an active forward thrusting of the hip on the right ("lift"), so that the traction effect on the throwing arm, and as a consequence on the 800 g (for men) and 600 g (for women) heavy javelin, increases greatly. **The trunk,** which is a central part of the whole-body extensor sling at the beginning of the movement – and this applies to all throwing and putting movements – **always precedes the throwing arm** in the sense of anticipating it **in order to,** at the right moment, **transfer the whole traction and extension force to the javelin** in the split-second throwing movement.

Only an inexperienced athlete would think that he or she can throw the javelin only with a movement of the arm. Only when he or she realizes that **three conditions must be fullfilled for a successful throw,** will he or she be able to attain the desired throwing distance. These three conditions are:

- a smooth, fast run-up,
- a pronounced arching of the whole body (during which the javelin is still held behind the hip, which has been brought forward and upward and
- a lifting at the moment of extension.

The throwing of the javelin requires, as a consequence, **great strength** in the trunk, and **great mobility** in the shoulder joint and shoulder girdle, in order to ensure the necessary propulsion of the javelin and the linear transfer of power at the moment of throwing. This is demonstrated in fig. 34.

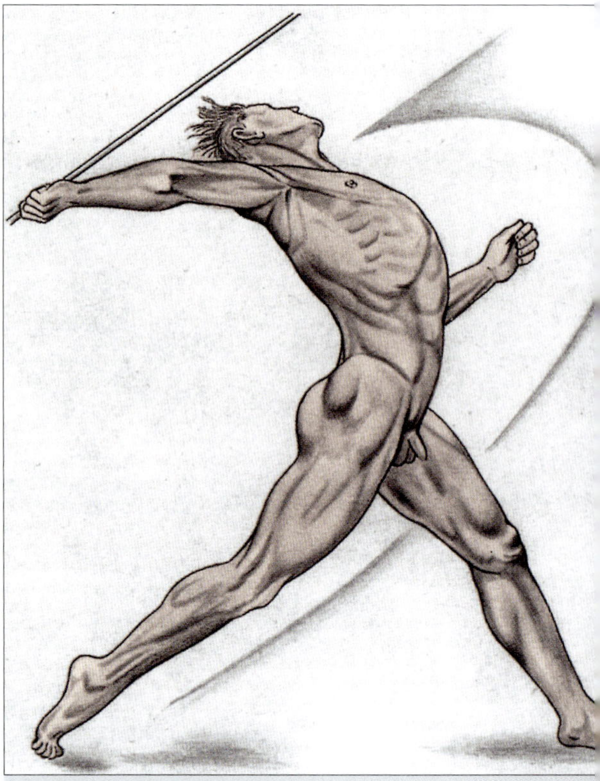

Fig. 34 Extensor sling over the whole body (tension of the bow) in a javelin thrower.

At this point we would like to make a brief digression from the actual course of the sling in order to present the diversity of the interplay of muscles. Precise observations have shown that the gluteus maximus with its fibres – as mentioned above – flows not only into the fascia thoracolumbalis on the same side but also into the fascia on the other side. The muscle thus continues into the latissimus dorsi on the other side of the body. In this way its effect on the knee joint, via the Maissiat band, and on the arm via the connection with the latissimus dorsi on the other side, increases. Because of the crossing-over of the two large muscle-tendon belts behind the centre of gravity of the body they also influence as **"guardians of equilibrium"** the position of the pelvis and the lumbar spine, and thus of the **whole body.**

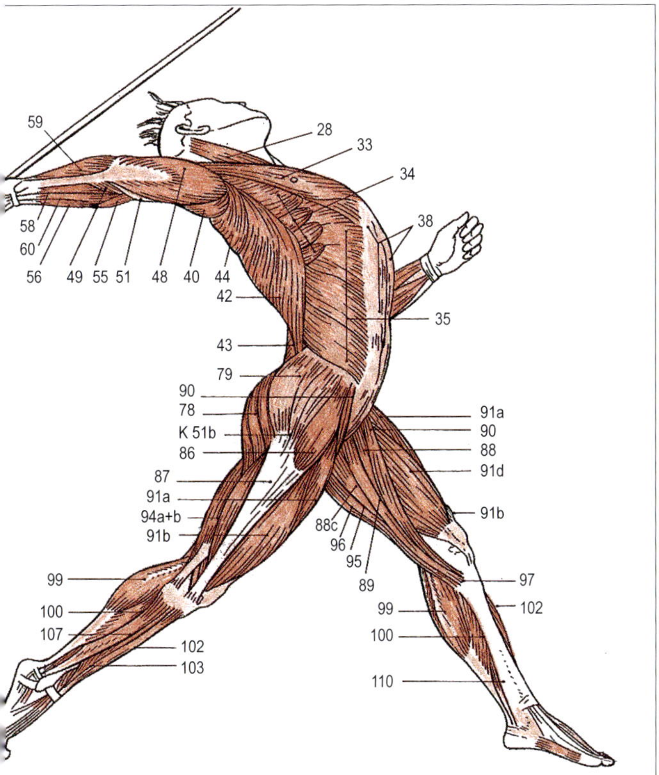

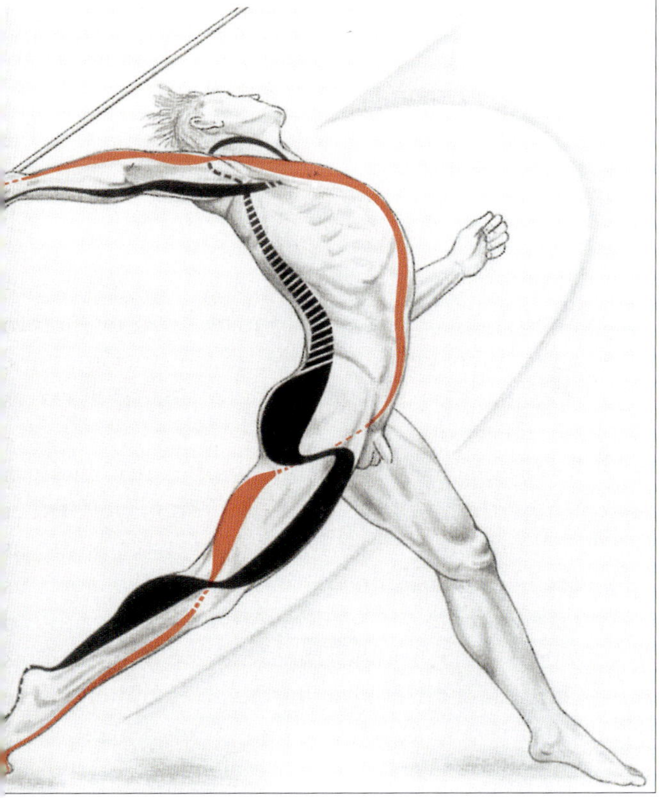

Muscles Fig. 34

28 Sternocleidomastoideus
33 Pectoralis major
34 Serratus anterior
35 Obliquus externus abdominis
38 Rectus abdominis
40 Supra- et infraspinatus
42 Latissimus dorsi
43 Fascia thoracolumbalis
44 Teres major
48 Triceps brachii
49 Anconeus
51 Brachialis
55 Brachioradialis
56 Extensor carpi radialis longus
58 Extensor carpi ulnaris
59 Flexor carpi ulnaris
60 Extensor digitorum
78 Gluteus maximus
79 Gluteus medius
86 Tensor fasciae latae
87 Tractus iliotibialis
88c Adductor magnus
89 Gracilis
90 Sartorius
91a Rectus femoris
91b Vastus lateralis
91d Vastus intermedius
94a Biceps femoris, caput longum
94b Biceps femoris, caput breve
95 Semimembranosus
96 Semitendinosus
97 Pes anserinus
99 Gastrocnemius
100 Soleus
102 Tibialis anterior
103 Extensor digitorum longus
107 Fibularis longus
110 Flexor digitorum longus

K51b Trochanter major

"These muscle-tendon strands which cross over from the arm to the knee are used by children who are sitting on a swing and trying to gain momentum. They hold their hands tightly on the ropes which hold the swing and bend their upper bodies against their legs, which are resting on the seat. In this way the buttocks are moved backwards. And now the long extended muscle belts contract; trunk and pelvis are gripped from behind and pressed forward. The gymnast who is hanging on the horizontal bar or swinging on the parallel bars, does much the same thing. The more the pelvis is flexed in all these positions, the greater is the extension of the gluteus maximus and the power with which he pushes the pelvis forward." (Hoepke, 1979)

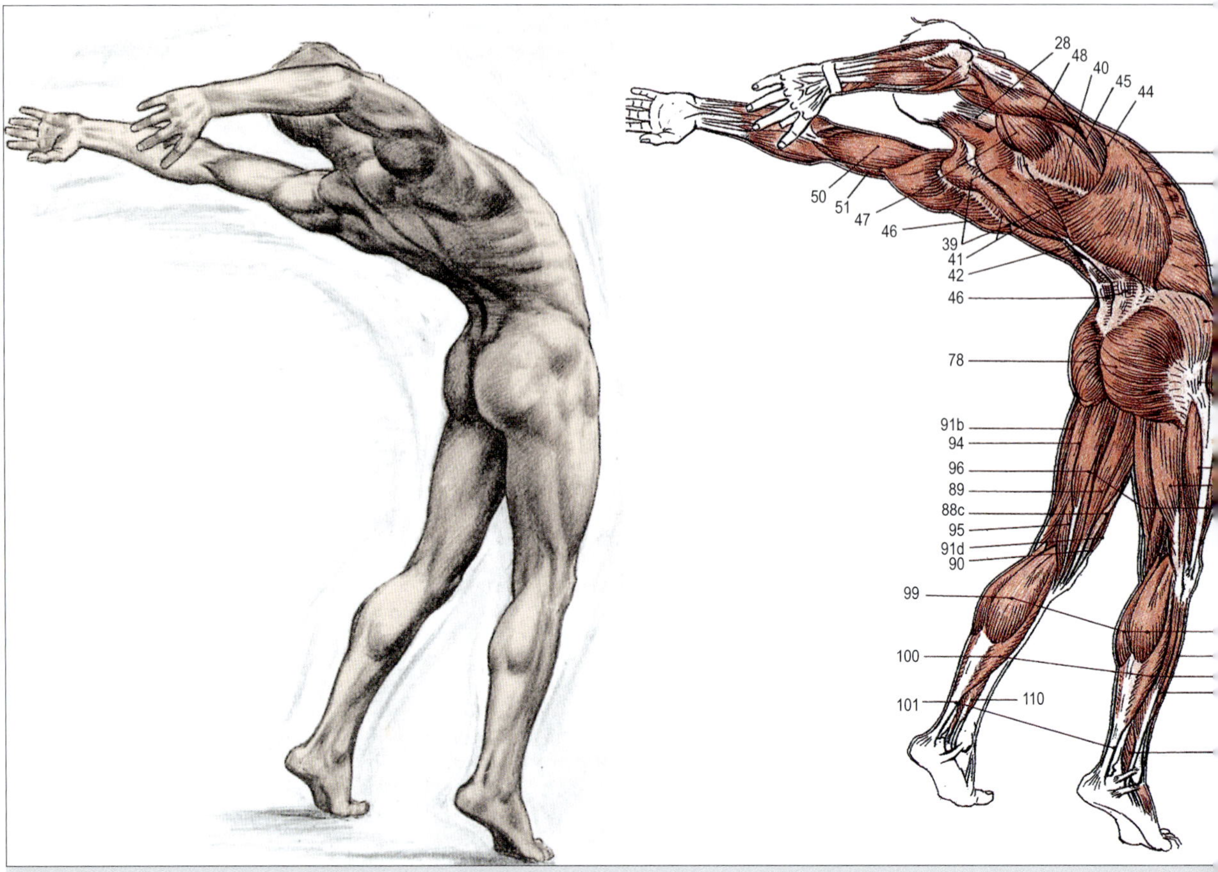

Fig. 35 Backwards overextension of the body in throwing a medicine ball.

Medicine-ball thrower

Fig. 35 shows the very powerful overextension of the whole body of a medicine-ball thrower. The 5 kg-heavy training ball has just been thrown with a backward sweep of the body. The extent to which especially this exercise is a **typical movement of the whole body,** can be seen from the illustration and from tables 4 and 5. This exercise can, among other things, be used in the rehabilitation of injuries of the trunk and the pelvis using balls of varying weight.

It is easy to see that the muscles of the arm and the shoulder joint for the extension of the arm at the shoulder joint (the corresponding antagonists are also shown for comparison) would not be sufficiently powerful to throw the medicine ball successfully.

This requires the recruitment of much larger muscle groups: the vertical utilization of the trunk muscles and the cooperation of the gluteus maximus and the latissimus dorsi on the other side, as shown in the illustration.

The sequence of movements of a medicine-ball thrower shows very clearly the great importance of the trunk as a weight-bearing and stable "pillar" of the body, and as the starting point of dynamic and static movements, as demonstrated in the athletes who use parallel bars, rings and the horizontal bar (fig. 81). With its great **muscle-power potential** the trunk is capable of functioning as an element which facilitates the preparation, acceleration and transfer within the whole-body muscle sling.

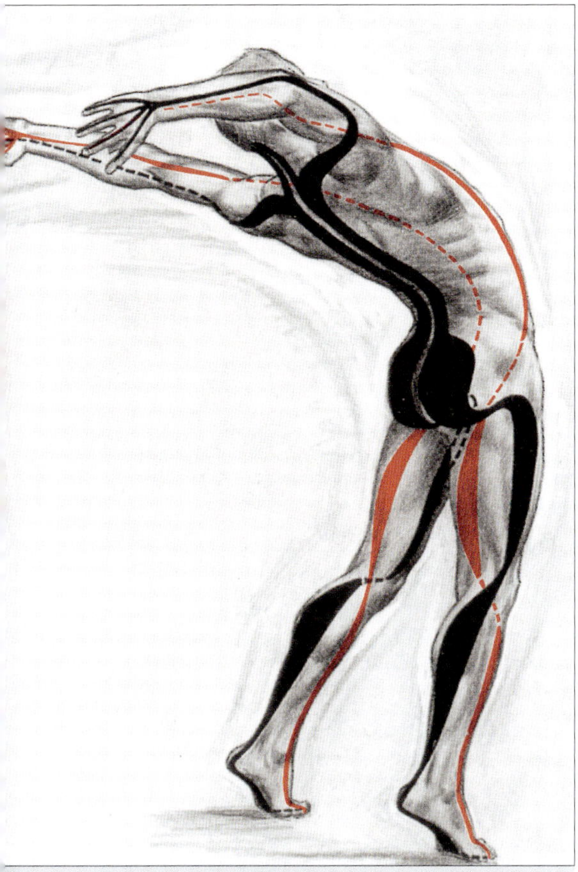

Muscles Fig. 35

28	Sternocleidomastoideus	**89**	Gracilis
33	Pectoralis major	**90**	Sartorius
34	Serratus anterior	**91b**	Vastus lateralis
35	Obliquus externus abdominis	**91d**	Vastus intermedius
		94	Biceps femoris
39	Trapezius	**95**	Semimembranosus
40	Supra- et infraspinatus	**96**	Semitendinosus
41	Rhomboideus major	**99**	Gastrocnemius
42	Latissimus dorsi	**99a**	Gastrocnemius, caput mediale
44	Teres major		
45	Teres minor	**99b**	Gastrocnemius, caput laterale
46	Erector spinae		
47	Deltoideus	**100**	Soleus
48	Triceps brachii	**101**	Tendo calcaneus
50	Biceps brachii	**103**	Extensor digitorum longus
51	Brachialis		
78	Gluteus maximus	**107**	Fibularis longus
79	Gluteus medius	**108**	Fibularis brevis
86	Tensor fasciae latae	**110**	Flexor digitorum longus
87	Tractus iliotibialis		
88c	Adductor magnus	**K51b**	Trochanter major

Table 4: Work potentials of the muscles which lift the upper arm upwards and backwards at the shoulder joint (extensors) by 107°, from 70° flexion to 37° extension.

	kg/m
Posterior deltoid	3.8
Subscapularis	0.9
Teres minor	0.4
Triceps, long head	6.8
Teres major	5.4
Latissimus dorsi, upper part	2.4
Latissimus dorsi, lower part	1.5
Pectoralis major, part of the abdominal fascia	0.1
All extensors	21.3

Table 5: Work potentials of the muscles which lift the upper arm forwards at the shoulder joint (flexors) by 107°, from 37° extension to 70° flexion.

	kg/m
Anterior deltoid	3.2
Medial deltoid	8.9
Supraspinatus	2.8
Infraspinatus	1.3
Subscapularis	0.9
Pectoralis major, clavicular part	1.9
Pectoralis major, sternal-costal part	2.8
Coracobrachialis	2.5
Biceps brachii, short head (at extended elbow)	1.7
Biceps brachii, long head	2.1
All flexors	28.1

Inappropriate strain and, in particular, a lifestyle which lacks movement, greatly impair the efficiency of the trunk and the spine by making them dysfunctional and unstable, and by increasing the risk of falls (with their consequences and lengthy stays in hospital). From a prophylactic, rehabilitation and functional-anatomical perspective, regular, age-adapted and power-orientated training of the whole body of the muscles shown in fig. 35 is of great importance for the dynamic stabilization of the central axial skeleton.

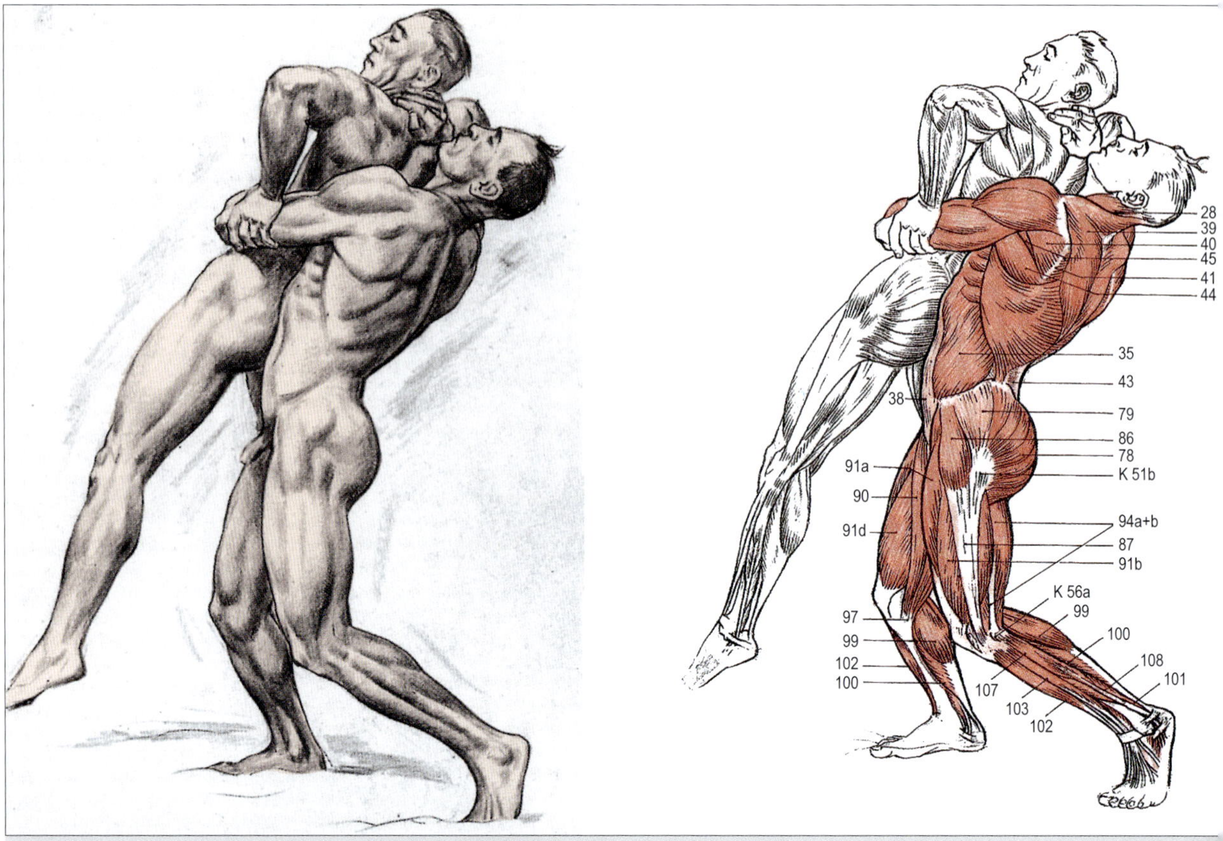

Fig. 36 Extensor sling over the whole of the body in standing combat in wrestling.

Wrestler (standing combat)

The next illustration (fig. 36), the wrestlers in standing combat, shows the main technique of Greco-Roman classical wrestling, the "throw over the chest", which is subdivided in four phases (which show the different ways in which power is applied):

- approaching the opponent and grabbing hold of him or her
- sudden shifting of the centre of gravity of the body, caused by lifting up the opponent from the ground and by explosive extension at the knee joint
- fast and powerful "abdominal push" forwards and upwards and extension of the trunk backwards ("hollowed-back tension") and
- sidewards turning and holding the opponent in a back-arch position.

In this style of wrestling, which is preferred by taller wrestlers, the holds are allowed only above the waistline, and down as far as the hip. In the second style of wrestling, **free-style wrestling,** which is preferred by shorter wrestlers, the whole body of the opponent, including the legs, which are used for defense and attack, is involved as the main target in combat.

Specific physical conditions are required in wrestling: his/her height should lie between 155 and 190 cm, depending on the weight categories in wrestling, and his/her average weight should be about 71.5 kg. Wrestlers are of the "metromorphic" and "lepto-metromorphic" type ("leptomorphic" = long and narrow; "metromorphic/mesomorphic" = above average muscular development). Particular individual physical proportions can facilitate or hinder the learning of specific traction and throwing techniques.

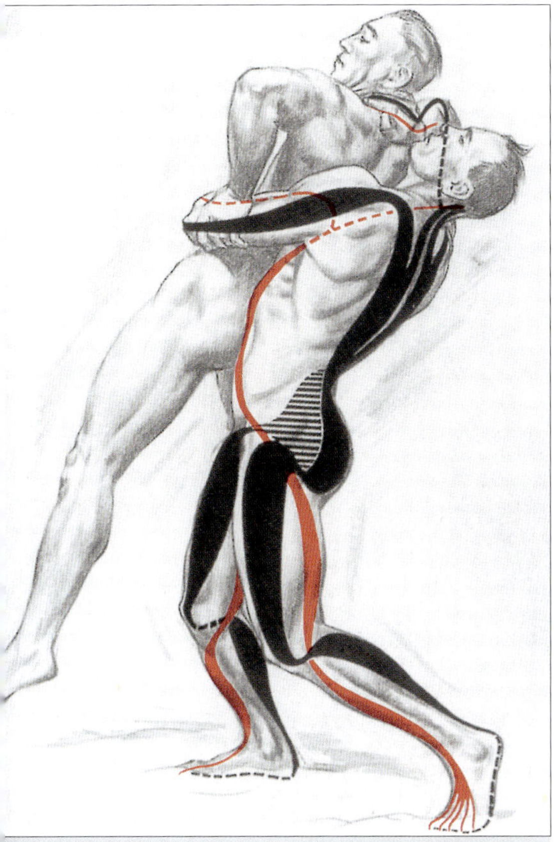

Muscles Fig. 36

- **28** Sternocleidomastoideus
- **35** Obliquus externus abdominis
- **38** Rectus abdominis
- **39** Trapezius
- **40** Supra- et infraspinatus
- **41** Rhomboideus major
- **43** Fascia thoracolumbalis
- **44** Teres major
- **45** Teres minor
- **78** Gluteus maximus
- **79** Gluteus medius
- **86** Tensor fasciae latae
- **87** Tractus iliotibialis
- **90** Sartorius
- **91a** Rectus femoris
- **91b** Vastus lateralis
- **91d** Vastus intermedius
- **94a** Biceps femoris, caput longum
- **94b** Biceps femoris, caput breve
- **97** Pes anserinus
- **99** Gastrocnemius
- **100** Soleus
- **101** Tendo calcaneus
- **102** Tibialis anterior
- **103** Extensor digitorum longus
- **107** Fibularis longus
- **108** Fibularis brevis

- **K51b** Trochanter major
- **K56a** Caput fibulae

The muscle extensor sling, which is the basis of these phases of movement, is shown on both sides of the body in the wrestler who is lifting his opponent in standing combat. The enormous power of the trunk, the arms and the legs is striking. This muscle extensor sling must work against the body-mass of the lifting wrestler and his active resistance in the technique and tactics of attack and defense. This requires a **larger proportion of fast-twitch fibres** in the skeletal muscles of wrestlers, which determines the rapid and explosive power specific to this sport discipline, and in the moment of a hold. In addition to the technical and tactical capabilities, this kind of power is crucial for success.

! "Explosive power" means the capability to mobilize as large a proportion as possible of the maximum available power-potential in the shortest possible time, in the specific circumstances of combat.

On the other hand, the extensor sling shows that it extends as far as the tips of the toes in order to make the accelerative path as long as possible. In addition, the extensor sling over the whole body is directly combined with the powerful use of the antagonists. As the **muscle sling is closed at both ends** (surface of the mat and the tightly held opponent), they switch their points of origin and insertion and thus no longer brake the course of the movement, but support it in a fast and powerful manner (as happens in the case of the powerful abdominal push). This principle will often be seen in the following sequences of movements, and underlies every successful throw (which happens unexpectedly and with very variable and coordinated use of muscles).

Wrestler (ground combat)

Muscles Fig. 37

- **28** Sternocleidomastoideus
- **35** Obliquus externus abdominis
- **38** Rectus abdominis
- **39** Trapezius
- **40** Supra- et infraspinatus
- **41** Rhomboideus major
- **42** Latissimus dorsi
- **43** Fascia thoracolumbalis
- **44** Teres major
- **45** Teres minor
- **47** Deltoideus
- **78** Gluteus maximus
- **79** Gluteus medius
- **86** Tensor fasciae latae
- **87** Tractus iliotibialis
- **90** Sartorius
- **91** Quadriceps femoris
- **91a** Rectus femoris
- **91b** Vastus lateralis
- **91d** Vastus intermedius
- **94** Biceps femoris, longum
- **94a** Biceps femoris, caput
- **94b** Biceps femoris, caput breve
- **97** Pes anserinus
- **99** Gastrocnemius
- **100** Soleus
- **101** Tendo calcaneus
- **102** Tibialis anterior
- **103** Extensor digitorum longus
- **107** Fibularis longus
- **108** Fibularis brevis

- **K51b** Trochanter major
- **K56a** Caput fibulae

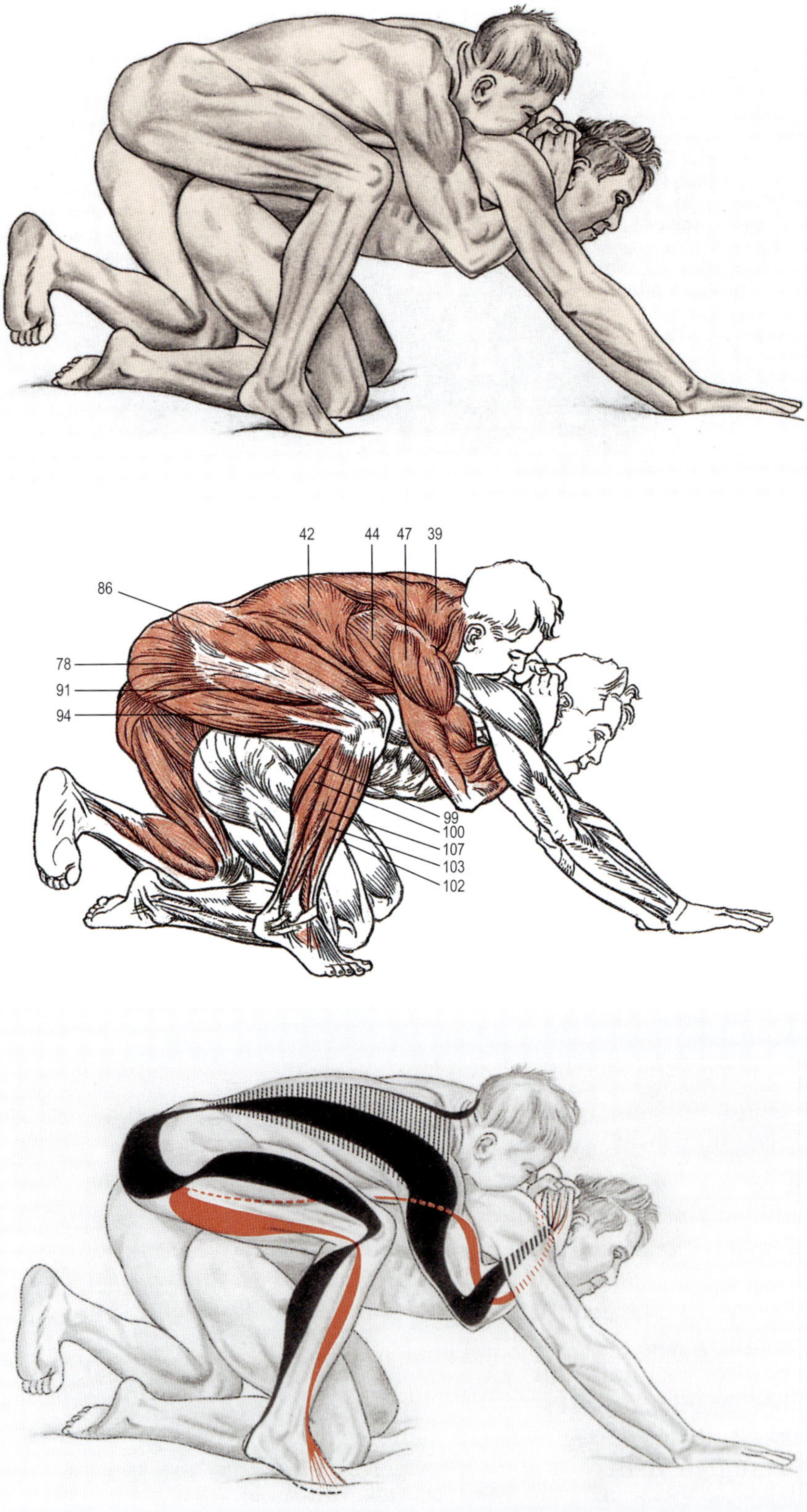

Fig. 37 Wrestling in ground combat. Look at the man on top and the varying strain put on the individual sections of the spine: flexion in the lumbar region, rotation in the thoracic region and extension or over-extension in the cervical section.

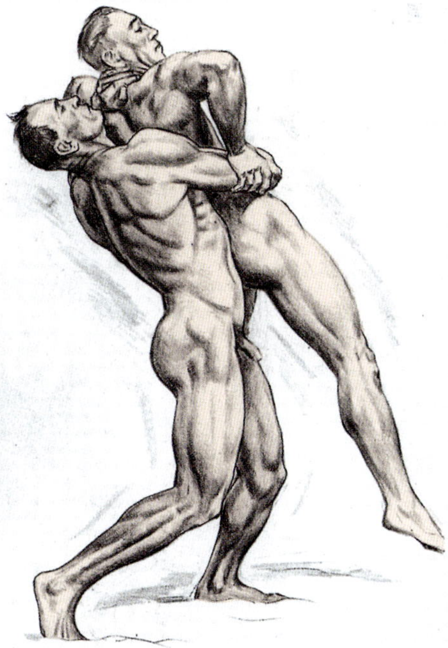

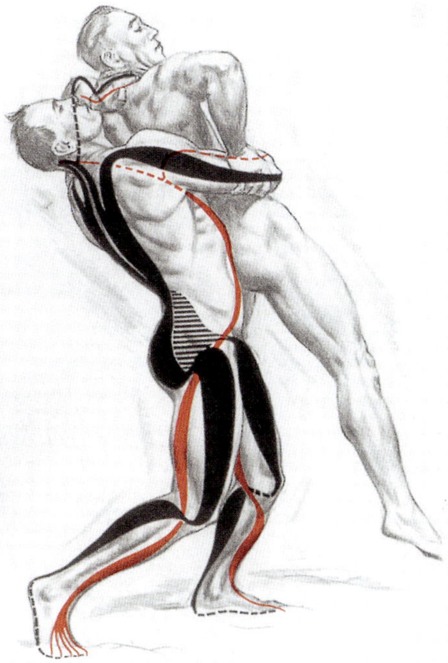

Fig. 38 Compare the naturalistic illustrations and the muscle slings of the wrestlers – ground combat and standing combat.

This applies also to another phase of wrestling, ground combat (fig. 37), in which one of the two wrestlers tries to break the "bridge position" of his opponent or to succeed by applying effective ground techniques which are given high scores. To do this he once again uses the muscle slings described above in applying rapid power, especially when forcefully lifting and pulling his opponent around. This capability makes it possible for the wrestler and judoka to use holds and throws rapidly and over a longer period of time. It should be mentioned here that, when the wrestler is held down in the "arched back" position, because of his over-extended cervical spine, his opponent is permitted in this situation – according to the rules – only to push him sideways.

The naturalistic illustration and the muscle drawing (fig. 38) should be used to revise and consolidate what has been learnt so far about the cooperation of agonists and antagonists, by comparing the two drawings, and to study the shifting movements of the individual muscles in a living person.

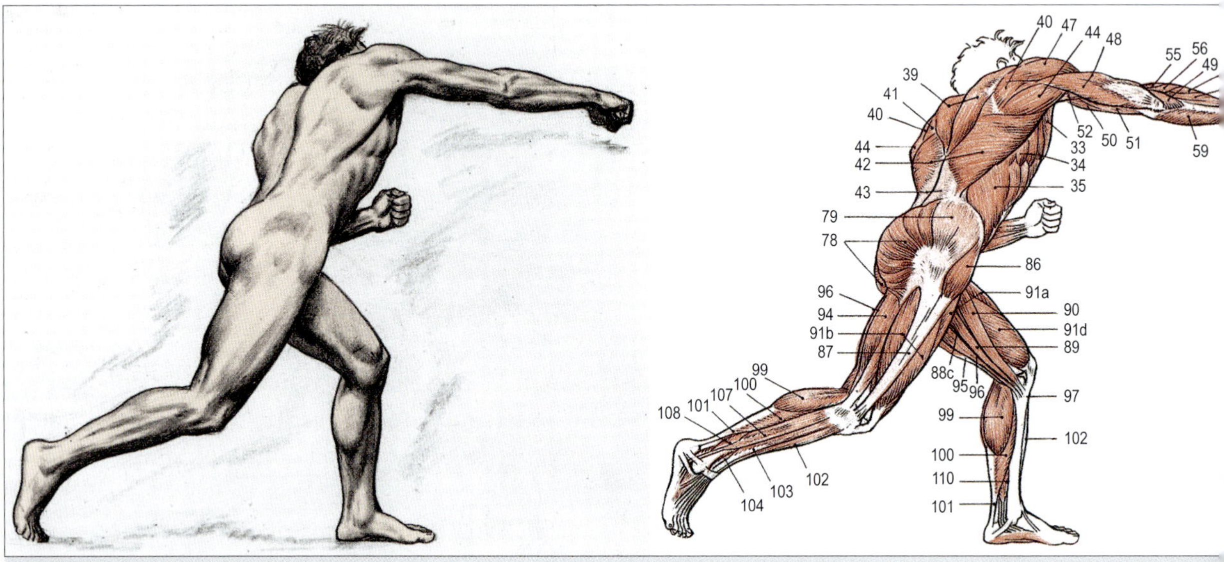

Fig. 39 Extensor sling over the whole body in a boxer throwing a right jab.

Boxer

Successful boxing requires not only great punching power and precision, but also great speed of reaction, punching and moving and the ability to anticipate movements of the legs, the arms and the trunk in order to be able to counter and avoid the opponent's sudden attacks. The **force impulse** of the first two capabilities in boxing are a result of 30 % of the maximum power application and 70 % of the maximum speed of movement. This demonstrates clearly that **this kind of sport is characterized by speed and power,** which are distinguished by a high degree of coordinative abilities. The boxer exhibits all these abilities when throwing a right jab (fig. 39).

This example was chosen to demonstrate the involvement of the whole body in the sequence of movements. The targeted jab is not only carried out by contraction of the muscles of the upper and lower arm, as a lay person would assume. The boxer puts his whole accelerated body mass and the great power of the muscles of his trunk, arms and legs into the punch. He "jumps" at his opponent, which can often be observed in the lower weight categories. This kind of movement can also be encountered in a similar form in fencing. If the punch misses its target, then the boxer runs the risk of falling, pulled forward by the momentum of his own body.

The extensor sling divides above the line of origin of the gluteus maximus so that one part (the one following the erector spinae) extends to the occiput, whereas the major portion of the power output is transferred, via the latissimus dorsi and the teres major, into the right upper extremity and ends in the fingers of the clenched fist.

Muscle strength and power are also essential components for physical performance. Muscle power is an important precondition for successfully carrying out very fast technical and tactical activities. If we try to define both terms, then **"strength"** signifies a muscle's ability to exert great force, whereas **"power"** signifies the explosive nature of the production of that force.

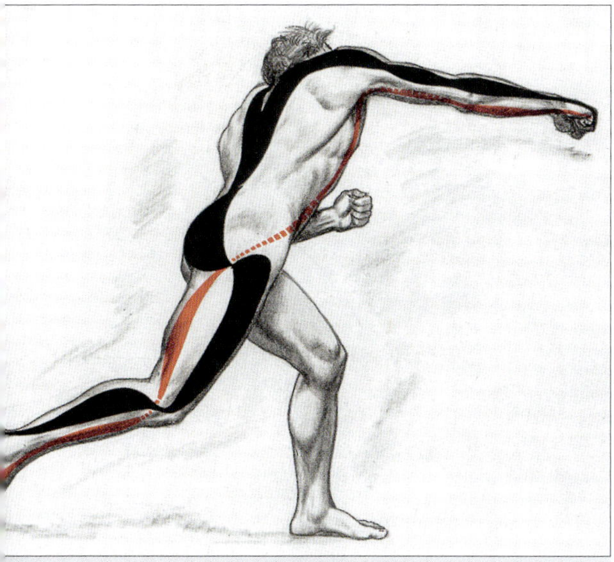

Muscles Fig. 39
33 Pectoralis major
34 Serratus anterior
35 Obliquus externus abdominis
39 Trapezius
40 Supra- et infraspinatus
41 Rhomboideus major
42 Latissimus dorsi
43 Fascia thoracolumbalis
44 Teres major
47 Deltoideus
48 Triceps brachii
49 Anconeus
50 Biceps brachii
51 Brachialis
52 Coracobrachialis
55 Brachioradialis
56 Extensor carpi radialis longus
57 Extensor carpi radialis brevis
59 Flexor carpi ulnaris
60 Extensor digitorum
78 Gluteus maximus
79 Gluteus medius
86 Tensor fasciae latae
87 Tractus iliotibialis
88c Adductor magnus
89 Gracilis
90 Sartorius
91a Rectus femoris
91b Vastus lateralis
91d Vastus intermedius
94 Biceps femoris
95 Semimembranosus
96 Semitendinosus
97 Pes anserinus
99 Gastrocnemius
100 Soleus
101 Tendo calcaneus
102 Tibialis anterior
103 Extensor digitorum longus
104 Extensor digitorum brevis
107 Fibularis longus
108 Fibularis brevis

Crucial factors for the **development of muscle power** are:

- the increase in the size of fast-twitch muscle fibres (hypertrophy)
- the high velocity of muscle contraction
- specific daily heavy-resistance power training
- the quality of coordinated, hierarchically ordered capabilities of spatial orientation, of kinesthetic differentiation, of reacting, of maintaining rhythm and balance and
- some physical preconditions and characteristics (see table 6).

Table 6: Selected body characteristics of participaters of Olympic Games in wrestling and boxing.

Body characteristics	Wrestling	Boxing
Body height/BH (cm)	170.0	169.3
Body mass/BM (kg)	71.3	63.1
Trunk length	52.2	51.3
Arm length	56.9	57.3
Leg length	77.7	78.1
Relative trunk length (%)	30.6	30.3
Relative arm length (%)	33.4	33.8
Relative leg length	45.7	46.3
BH/BM Relation cm/g	12.44	12.91

Boxers have, in comparison to wrestlers, a shorter trunk and relatively long extremities. The most important difference lies in the increased athletic shaping of the body. Wrestlers and boxers have an above-average muscular development and are athletically built or thin (mesomorphic to lepto-/mesomorphic type).

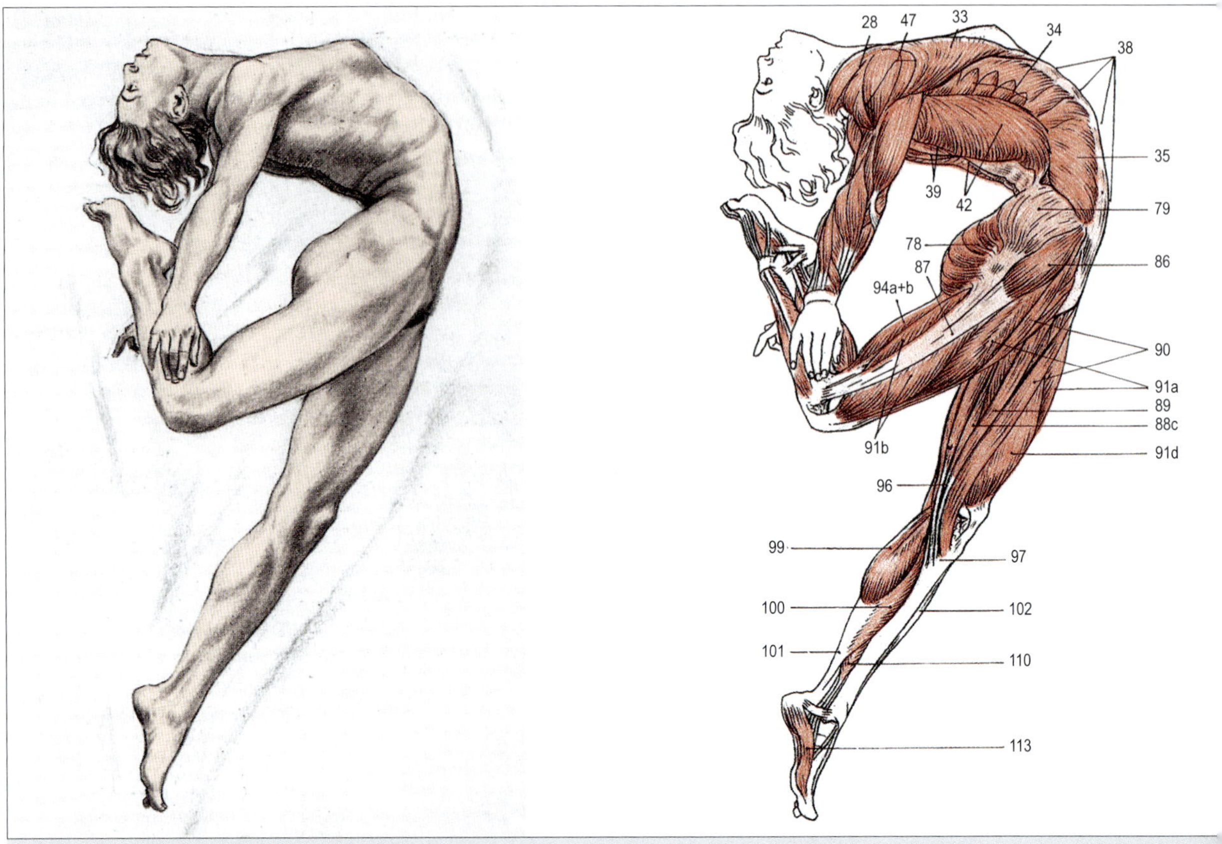

Fig. 40 Extensor sling over the whole body in a gymnast.

Gymnast

In women's gymnastics (fig. 40) there is, worldwide, a continuous increase in technically demanding, attractive movement elements which make great demands on the speed of general movement and special coordination, and on the vestibular and kinaesthetic system for differentiated perception of position and movement. They are a necessary condition of the reliable performance of whole-body movements which involve high rotational speed. The drawing of the gymnast shows that the contractile strength of the extensor sling over the whole body and the extension ability of the antagonists are of major importance for this sport discipline as well (which is counted among the technical disciplines, such as diving, ice-skating and ball-room dancing), so that the exercises can be performed accurately and completed precisely.

It is worth noting the great mobility and indeed **hypermobility** (in doing the splits on the ground, in standing or jumping) of the shoulder, hip and ankle joints and the **overextension of the spine at the lumbo-sacral transition.** There is a new aspect to be considered with regard to the right leg of the gymnast: the course of the sling in which the flexors of the lower leg (the biceps femoris, the semitendinosus and semimembranosus muscles), which lie on the back of the thigh, are united with the plantar flexors (the gastrocnemius and the soleus).
Table 7 shows the power and speed of the flexors of the lower leg at the knee joint in this sequence of movements.

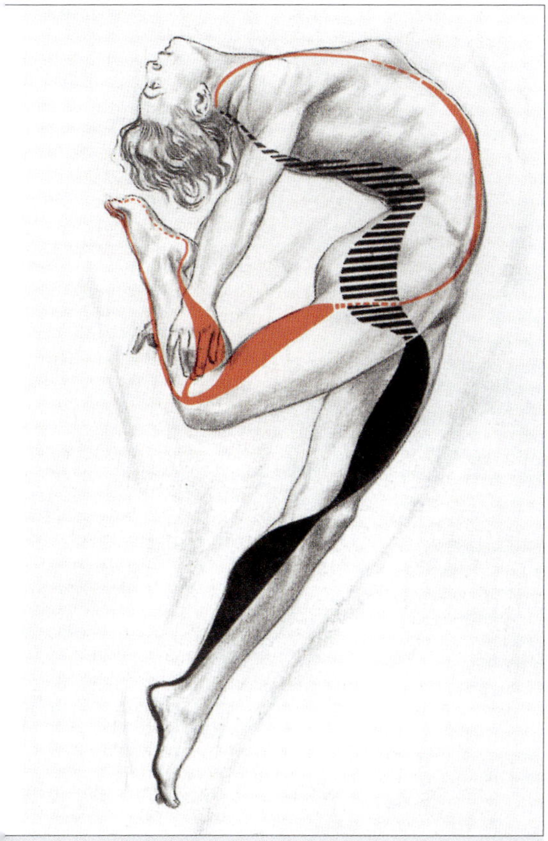

Muscles Fig. 40

28 Sternocleidomastoideus
33 Pectoralis major
34 Serratus anterior
35 Obliquus externus abdominis
38 Rectus abdominis
39 Trapezius
42 Latissimus dorsi
47 Deltoideus
78 Gluteus maximus
79 Gluteus medius
86 Tensor fasciae latae
87 Tractus iliotibialis
88c Adductor magnus
89 Gracilis
90 Sartorius
91a Rectus femoris
91b Vastus lateralis
91d Vastus intermedius
94a Biceps femoris, caput longum
94b Biceps femoris, caput breve
96 Semitendinosus
97 Pes anserinus
99 Gastrocnemius
100 Soleus
101 Tendo calcaneus
102 Tibialis anterior
110 Flexor digitorum longus
113 Abductor hallucis

'able 7: Work potential of the flexors of the lower leg at the knee joint.

	kg/m
Sartorius	2.3
Gracilis	3.1
Semimembranosus	16.8
Semitendinosus	13.2
Biceps femoris, long and short head	10.3
All flexors	**45.7**

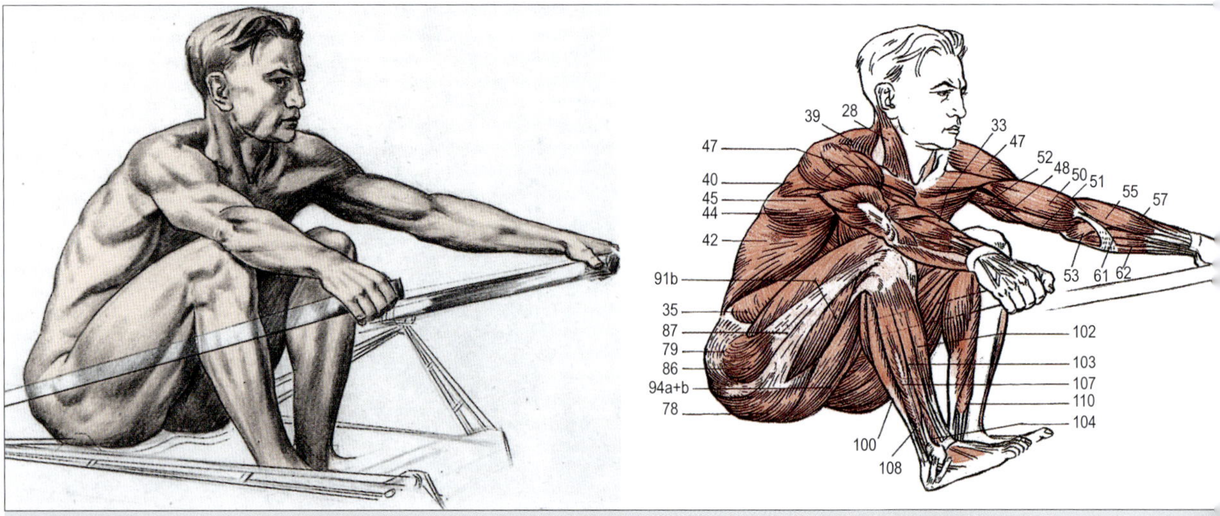

Fig. 41 Extensor sling over the whole of the body of a rower (anterior-lateral view).

Rower

One of the most demanding, cyclical (rhythmically repeated) sequences of movements – as far as the physical condition of the athlete is concerned – is rowing (fig. 41 and 42). The power and power endurance capabilities of the rower with an average weight of 98 kg and a slim and athletic physique are the crucial conditions for great competitive performance. This becomes immediately clear if you consider that the best high-performance rowers generate in the middle of their course (on average per stroke) a power performance of 490 N and at the start 784 N, and that the race over 2000 metres requires approximately 200–240 strokes. The rower must cover this distance – depending on the type of boat and on the weather – in 5:30–7:30 min in a virtual steady-state by means of **aerobic** work ("stamina") in order to achieve, in the final 500 meters over 1:30 min ("final spurt"), the maximum final speed of the boat by means of **anaerobic** work.

This is reflected in the large strong muscles which unite to form a powerful extensor sling. If we look at the naturalistic drawing, the muscles of the extensor sling of the lower extremity can be clearly seen in fig. 41:

- the gluteus maximus,
- the quadriceps femoris,
- the gastrocnemius with
- the underlying soleus,

as well as parts of the superficial dorsal muscles, especially the anterior margin of the latissimus dorsi and the teres major, which bulge prominently from below the body surface.

The most important muscles in the drawing which are most active in the sequence of movements of the rower on his or her sliding seat are (fig. 41):

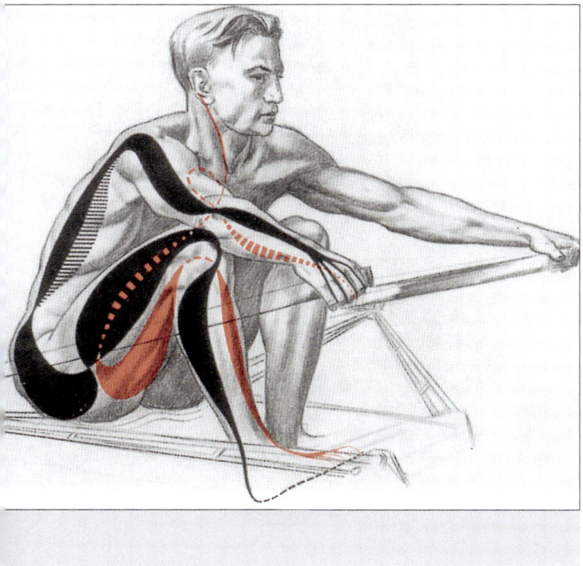

Muscles Fig. 41

28 Sternocleidomastoideus
33 Pectoralis major
35 Obliquus externus abdominis
39 Trapezius
40 Supra- et infraspinatus
42 Latissimus dorsi
44 Teres major
45 Teres minor
47 Deltoideus
48 Triceps brachii
50 Biceps brachii
51 Brachialis
52 Coracobrachialis
53 Pronator teres
55 Brachioradialis
57 Extensor carpi radialis brevis
61 Flexor carpi radialis
62 Flexor digitorum superficialis
78 Gluteus maximus
79 Gluteus medius
86 Tensor fasciae latae
87 Tractus iliotibialis
91b Vastus lateralis
94a Biceps femoris, caput longum
94b Biceps femoris, caput breve
100 Soleus
102 Tibialis anterior
103 Extensor digitorum longus
104 Extensor digitorum brevis
107 Fibularis longus
108 Fibularis brevis
110 Flexor digitorum longus

- the rectus abdominis and the iliopsoas, for the rhythmical forward roll of the trunk,
- the long and short deep dorsal muscles (erector spinae), for the backwards movement of the trunk,
- the gluteus maximus,
- the quadriceps femoris and
- the muscles of the calf: the gastrocnemius and the soleus.

It should be taken into consideration that the activity of the extensors of the trunk and the lower extremities when rowing a stroke ("water work") is preceded by **an intensive pre-extension** of these muscles – as can be seen from the whole posture which the rower adopts at the very moment of pulling back the blades. As opposed to rowing in a fixed seat and to paddling in a canoe, where the legs function only as stabilizers, the **powerful extension of the legs which do most of the work in rowing on a moveable seat** changes the initial angle of the knee joint from 60° to 150–160° at the end of a stroke. It is for this reason that signs of fatigue after intensive training or running are felt more in the muscles of the legs and hip joint than in the muscles of the arms.

That the main work in rowing has to be done by the legs has already been proved by the power measurements (hand pressure, contraction of dorsal and arm muscles) made by Bethe and Fischer (1929) in participants in the Olympic Games in Amsterdam (1928). These findings were confirmed by Daireaux and Pottier (1982), among others, with their electromyographic investigation of representative muscles in rowing. The extensor muscles of the lower extremity showed the highest activity ratings.

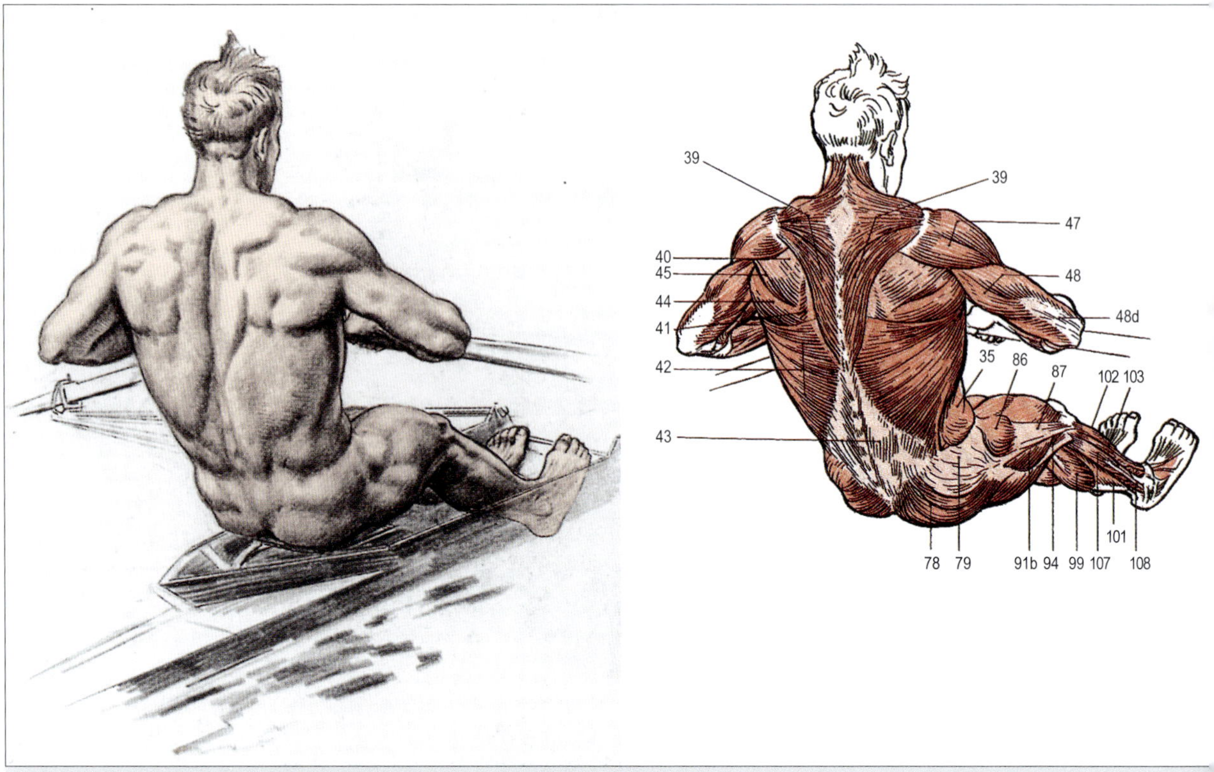

Fig. 42 Extensor sling over the whole of the body of a rower (seen from behind).

The naturalistic view of the second illustration of the rower (fig. 42) shows the powerfully developed and contracted dorsal muscles. Among the muscles of the superficial extensive dorsal muscles the following are particularly prominent:

- the trapezius, and while rowing a stroke
- the latissimus dorsi together with
- the teres major.

In the illustration showing the slings the powerful development of the extensor muscles of the lower extremity is particularly noticeable.

What unfortunately cannot been seen in fig. 41 and 42 is the **interplay between the gluteus maximus and the iliopsoas,** which has been omitted for the sake of clarity. Nonetheless this cooperation should be mentioned (fig. 43), as the iliopsoas, with the rectus abdominis, is responsible in rowing for bringing the trunk forward – after having been greatly extended at the end of a stroke – so that the rower can put the blades into the water far behind his or her body. After this the extensor sling which runs from head to foot – after being greatly extended by the preceding flexion of the trunk – pushes the pelvis forward, straightens up the trunk and extends the whole body.

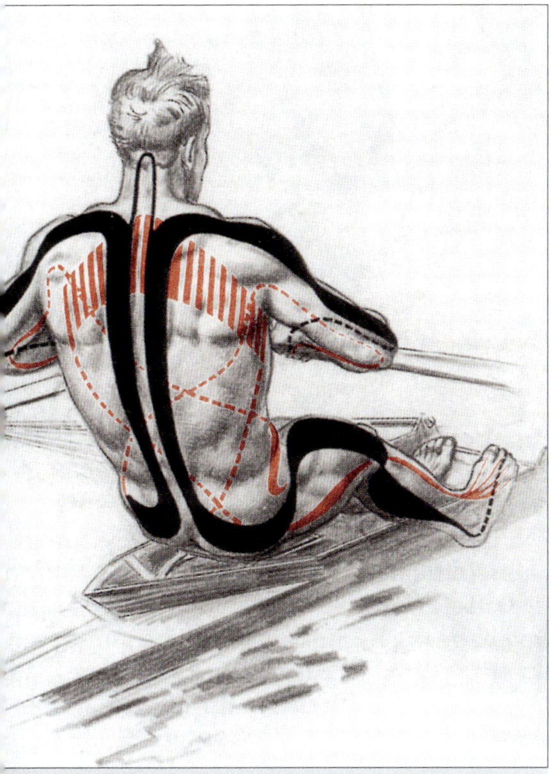

Muscles Fig. 42

35 Obliquus externus abdominis
39 Trapezius
40 Supra- et infraspinatus
41 Rhomboideus major
42 Latissimus dorsi
43 Fascia thoracolumbalis
44 Teres major
45 Teres minor
47 Deltoideus
48 Triceps brachii
48d Tendon of triceps brachii
78 Gluteus maximus
79 Gluteus medius
86 Tensor fasciae latae
87 Tractus iliotibialis
91b Vastus lateralis
94 Biceps femoris
99 Gastrocnemius
101 Tendo calcaneus
102 Tibialis anterior
103 Extensor digitorum longus
107 Fibularis longus
108 Fibularis brevis

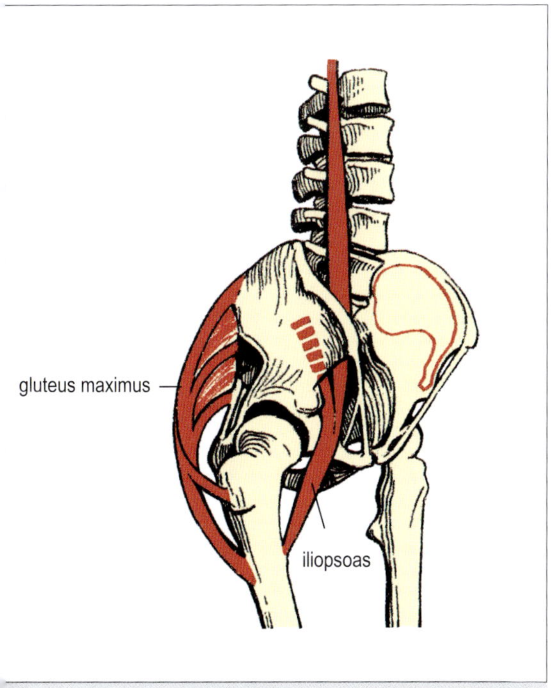

g. 43 Interplay between the gluteus maximus and iliopsoas. is interplay plays an important part, not only in sports, but also erveryday movements (climbing stairs), which would not be ssible without an intact interplay.

Lesion-prone weak point: lumbo-sacral transition

Strength performance, as already mentioned, is achieved above all by systematic weight training (with increasing weights). For this reason the sports physician and the trainer share the responsibility of looking for opportunities to further increase or decrease the load on the spine, and particularly on the lumbo-sacral transition (Cotta and Krahl 1980, Steinbrück 1982, Tittel 1981), which is often described as the "lesion-prone weak point of the spine". The lumbo-sacral transition is a feature of the human axial skeleton. It forms an open angle posteriorly of 142° (in men) and 144° (in women) between the lumbar spine and the sacral bone (fig. 44), where 70–75 % of the extension and over-extension of the lumbar spine takes place. The various functions of the lumbo-sacral transition make it necessary for it **to be as stable as possible and as flexible as necessary.**

This necessarily gives rise to the question of the capacity of the lumbo-sacral transition to bear the load and transfer part of the load to other structures. This is important above all when its static, mechanical and neural tasks overlap. This can be observed, for example, when there is **a decrease of stability in favour of an increase of mobility in this region.** This problem, which athletes, and those who look after them, have to deal with on a daily basis, is illustrated by the following analyses of various movements in sport from a functional-anatomical point of view.

The lumbo-sacral transition, which is put under great strain by the upright gait, by jumping and by lifting heavy weights carries out the tasks mentioned below, first by means of the **specific structure of the joint connection** formed by the articular processes of the sacral bone, which are located more anteriorly, and those of the 5th lumbar vertebra. This joint, often regarded as part of a "telescope", is put under strain by pressure (through axial compressive and crushing forces) and by pulling and shearing. **The articular connection functions** in this context like "ratchets" which **stop the lumbar spine slipping forward and practically prevent lateral inclination and rotation.**

Secondly, the ligaments and muscles have a crucial effect on the lumbo-sacral transition. When load is transferred from the trunk towards the lumbo-sacral

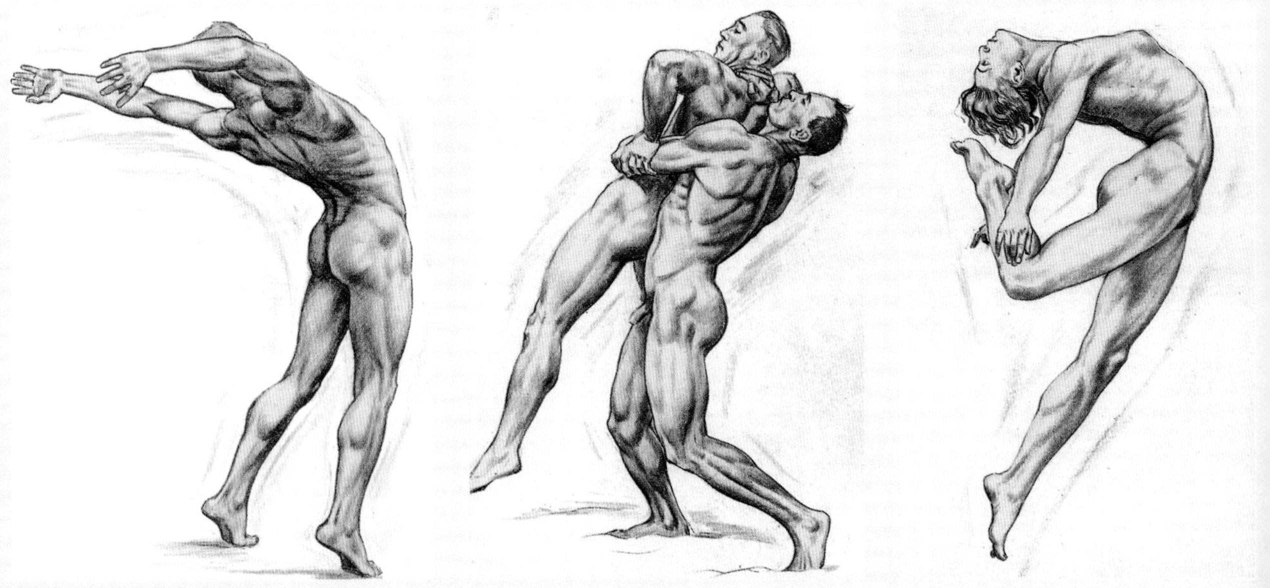

Fig. 44 Extension and overextension of the lumbar spine.

transition → sacro-iliac joints → pelvis (including the symphysis) → hip joints (fig. 45), there is a strong ligamental traction, the direction of which shows the main pathways of the load.

- In this way the **ilio-femoral ligament,** which is the strongest ligament in the whole body, prevents retroversion of the pelvis beyond 15–18° and is supported partly by the rectus femoris. This position is described as "stable pelvic inclination" in which the weight of the trunk is mainly borne by this ligament. This position makes it possible **to maintain a comfortable "resting posture"** while the "taut posture" is secured by muscles.
- Some other strong ligaments should be mentioned here: the **sacro-tuberal ligament** and the **sacro-spinal ligament** (fig. 45), which stop the sacral bone from slipping backwards when it is transferring the load.
- The **ilio-lumbar ligament** which inhibits the lateral movement of both of the lowest lumbar vertebrae.

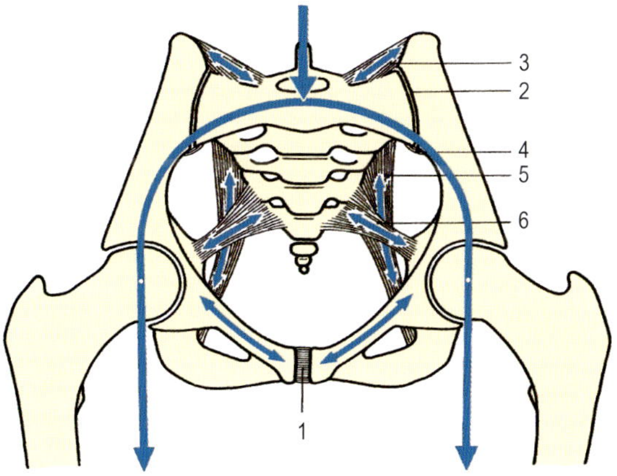

1 Symphysis
2 Sacro-iliac joint
3 Posterior sacro-iliac ligaments and interosseal sacro-iliac ligaments
4 Anterior sacro-iliac ligaments
5 Sacro-tuberal ligament
6 Sacro-spinal ligament

Fig. 45 Semi-schematized illustration of the curved construction of the pelvis and the main distribution of load from the lumbar spine to the sacroiliacal joints and to the acetabular roof (joint socket) on both sides. Top arrow = the weight of the trunk pressing on the pelvis; other arrows = strain on ligaments or bones from differing loads.

Because of this ligamental system and its close co-operation with the abdominal and spinal muscles, as well as with the contractors and extensors of the leg at the hip joint, the **lumbo-sacral transition is protected from extreme movements.**

This also has an effect on the hyaline joint cartilage and the wedge-shaped intervertebral disc between the last lumbar vertebra and the sacral bone.

Conclusions can be drawn about the inter-relationship between the lumbo-sacral transition and the inclination of the pelvis, which is limited posteriorly by the already mentioned iliofemoral ligament. This determines the posterior deflection of the lumbo-sacral transition, whereas it is variable in the anterior direction. If you compare extreme anterior and posterior movements with one another you notice that the angle formed by the lumbo-sacral transition increases if the angle of inclination of the pelvis decreases. Hence the spine can compensate for the movements of the pelvis with the help of the ligamental and muscular system already described.

As a result there can be relatively small shifts in the total body mass:

- The iliopsoas, the sartorius and the rectus femoris cause an **anterior inclination** of the pelvis (= lordotic curvature of the lumbar spine),
- The gluteus maximus, the biceps femoris, the semitendinosus and membranosus muscles cause a **posterior inclination** of the pelvis.

In other words: all the other parts of the axial skeleton change accordingly, starting with the lumbo-sacral transition, while the transition itself ensures the maintenance of the centre of gravity of the body in a "labile equilibrium".

Biomechanical analyses (Grok, Baumann, Thöss 1969; Wirehead 1984) have shown that the axial static load on the lumbo-sacral transition in a person holding a weight of 25 kg, when the trunk is inclined forwards and the legs are extended, comes to 480 kp, a load which increases by 200 kg and a trunk mass of 60 kg to 1090 kp. For this reason it is generally recommended that the person lifting the weight stands in such a way that the arm functioning as the outer lever (the distance from the lumbo-sacral transition to the centre of gravity of the body and to the weight to be lifted) is as short as possible. This means that **the load should be lifted close to the body with a straight back** (fig. 46).

By means of this lifting technique, which has to be learned at an early stage and which ensures a greater arm leverage and a shorter distance between spine and lever arm, the axial pressure caused by the weight is evenly distributed over the total surface of the vertebrae and intervertebral discs. This results in a significant reduction of load on the lumbo-sacral transition, which is to be taken into consideration in weight training.

For this lifting technique it is necessary to develop a strong extensor muscle sling in the lower extremity (fig. 46 and fig. 47), which makes it possible to stand up from a crouching position.

Deep inhalation and the tight closure of all the orifices of the abdomen and the thorax (especially the glottis) and the associated increase of intra-abdominal pressure for a few seconds make it easier to snatch the weight from the floor. At the same time the pressure within the intervertebral discs drops temporarily by more than 60 %.

Weightlifters, javelin throwers, discus throwers and shot-putters apply this knowledge and support the function of the abdominal muscles by wearing a leather belt around the waist, which becomes broader towards the back and which they put on immediately before the challenging task is about to be performed.

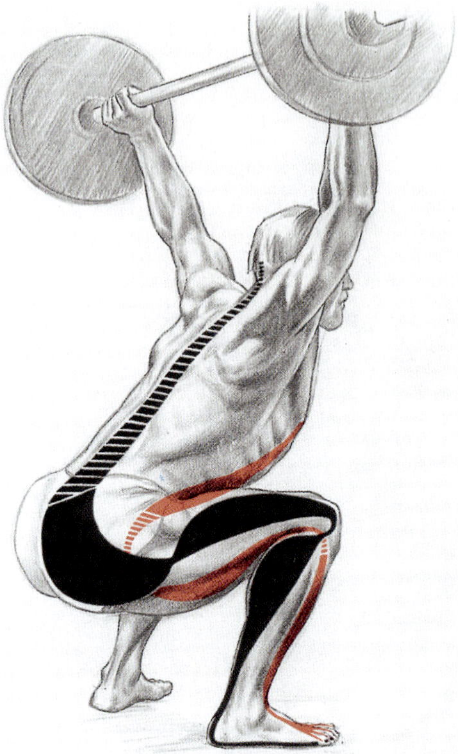

Fig. 46 Straight back and strong extensor muscles in a weight-lifter.

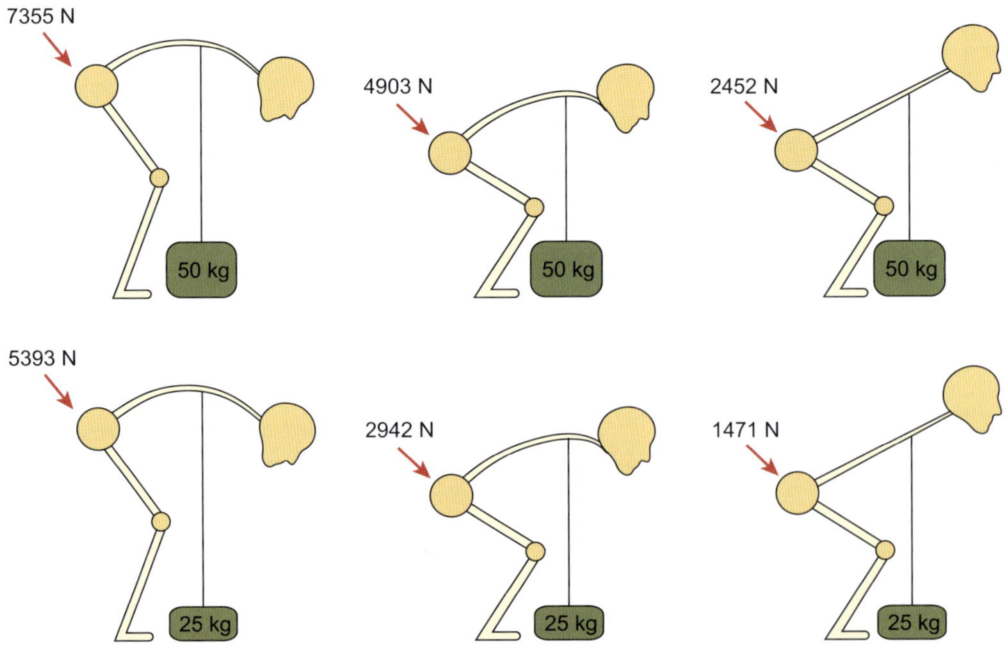

Fig. 47 Extremely different forces exerted on the lumbo-sacral transition when using a defective or a correct lifting technique (close to the body with a straight back).

Weightlifter

After these preliminary remarks, which will increase our understanding of the analysis of the following sequence of movements, we can turn to weightlifting (fig. 46 and fig. 47), and in particular the discipline of the "push". **The push consists of two phases:** after pulling the barbell upwards (which is 2.20 m long and loaded with plates weighing 0.5–25 kg), with the hands set wide apart, from the ground in a single pull up to the chest and from there to the shoulders **(pulling phase)**; the arms are regrouped from a pulling to a supporting position and there is a fast active lowering of the body until the knee is bent at an angle of 40° (lunge or squatting position). Further lowering of the body and the barbell is slowed down by means of a maximum contraction of the extensor muscles of the knee and hip as well as those of the elbow. This is the **braking phase** (as shown in the illustration) which requires mobility at the hip and the ankle joints, so that a low and stable squatting position is possible, and which makes great demands on the maintenance of body equilibrium. The muscles just mentioned develop, on the barbell, a strength which can increase to 170 % of the barbell's weight. At this point the athlete straightens up, developing the maximum power of the extensors of the hip, knee and upper ankle joints (tables 8–10) from a squatting position against the weight of the barbell to reach an extended standing position.

Thus in the two-arm push three clearly distinct capabilities can be distinguished which lift, hold and brake large to maximum weights:

- fast power to lift weights suddenly
- braking power and
- maximum power capability.

Each of these is characterized by a high level of functioning of the sensomotoric control system and requires, at muscle-cell level, the activation of as many motor units as possible to release maximum energy in the shortest possible time.

The stability of the body of the athlete and the maintenance of static and dynamic postural control are increased during the sequence of movements by the position of the feet and broad-based position of the legs (= extension of the supporting base) and by the flexion of the knee and the hip (= shortening of the distance between the centre of gravity of the body and the supporting base).

In the naturalistic illustration (fig. 48) the shaping of the body surface by the powerful extensor sling can be seen. The tensor fasciae latae is prominent as an oval-to-round bulging muscle. The main work for the initial phase of the straightening-up process is done by the quadriceps femoris (as can be seen in tables 8–10). In this it is supported by the gastrocnemius and soleus and – in order to push the pelvis forward, straighten up the spine, extend the hip joint and lift the trunk against the force of

Table 8: Work potential of the extensors of the thigh at the hip joint.

	kg/m
Contribution of the gluteus maximus to the fascia lata	20.3
Adductor femoris brevis	1.4
Adductor femoris magnus	22.2
Gracilis	1.0
Semimembranosus	18.7
Semitendinosus	7.7
Biceps femoris, long head	5.6
Gluteus maximus	43.3
Gluteus medius	11.7
Gluteus minimus	2.1
Piriformis	1.0
All extensors (including the obturatorius externus and the quadratus femoris)	135.0

Table 9: Work potential of the extensors of the lower leg at the knee joint.

	kg/m
Rectus femoris	23.4
Vastus lateralis Vastus medialis Vastus intermedius	118.6
Tensor fasciae latae	0.8
All extensors	142.8

Table 10: Work potential of the plantar flexors at the upper ankle joint.

	kg/m
Gastrocnemius, medial and lateral head	9.0
Soleus	7.4
Flexor digitorum longus	0.4
Tibialis posterior	0.4
Fibularis longus	0.4
Fibularis brevis	0.3
Flexor hallucis longus	0.9
All plantar flexors	18.8

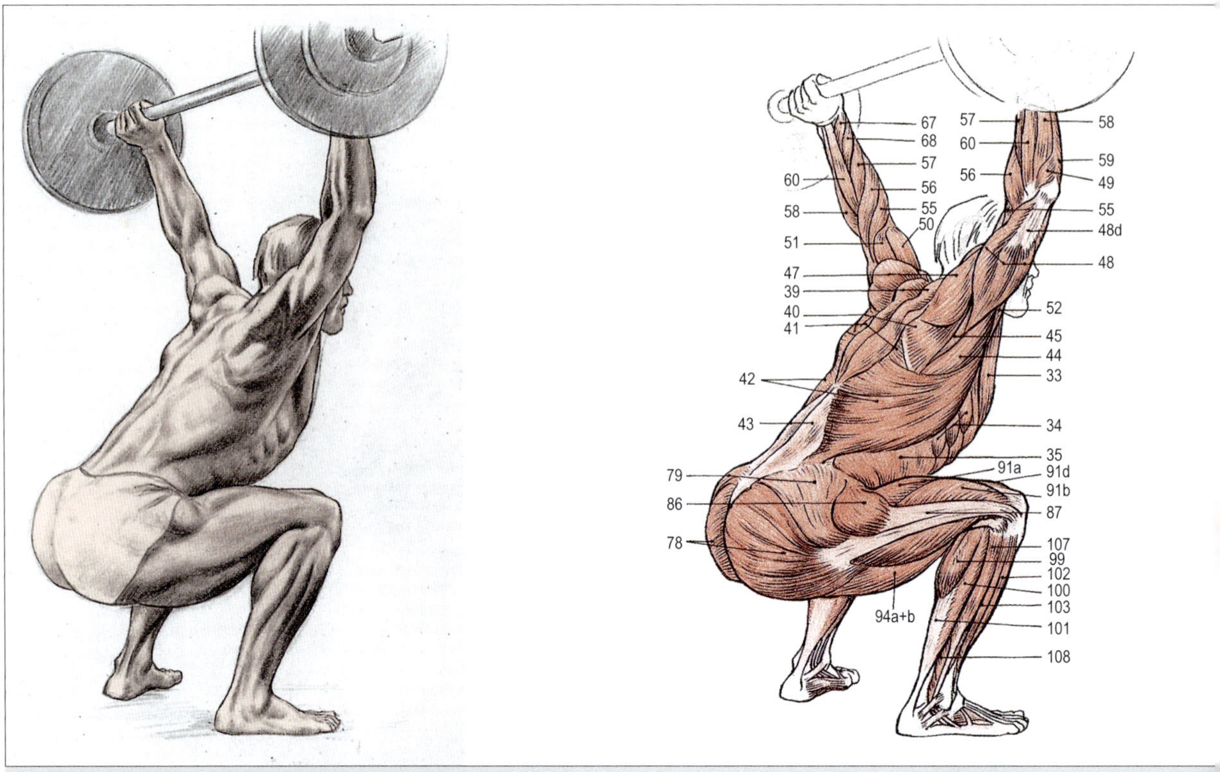

Fig. 48 Extensor slings over the whole body in a weightlifter during the push.

gravity – by the gluteus maximus and medius and by the extremely contracted muscles of the anterior lower leg and of the posterior thigh and by the abdominal muscles.

The extension muscle sling receives this support in the phase which directly precedes full extension (which can be observed in rowing and cycling where the feet and the pelvis are fixated: **closed sling** in cycling (pedal – saddle [pelvis] – handle bars) and in rowing (steering board [feet] – seat [pelvis] – firm hold of the oar). The **previous "antagonists",** when the pelvic girdle and the feet are fixated, **become,** for a short time, **"synergists" of the extensor muscles.** This makes it clear that the activity of the muscles running from the back of the thigh to the knee joint is always determined by the initial position of the section of the skeleton which lies cranially (which is the origin of the muscle group) and of the section which lies caudally. This example shows yet again that there is no predetermined and in every circumstance constant activity of the agonists as opposed to the antagonists.

By means of surface electromyography, which provides quantitative information about the muscle tension and duration of activity, it has been possible to show that during the push it is above all the **gastrocnemius and the iliocostalis** which show very high activity, whereas, during the balancing and fixation of the barbell in the broad-based squatting position and during the straightening-up phase, it is the **quadriceps femoris, the iliocostalis, the trapezius as well as the deltoid muscle** – and this is often overlooked – which have very high activity ratings.

Without the powerful contraction of the **deltoid muscle** (fig. 49) it would be impossible to hold the barbell steady above the head. It prevents the barbell from slipping away, which would inevitably lead to an elongation of the weight-bearing lever and thus to the need to use additional forces to bring the sequence of movements to a proper conclusion.

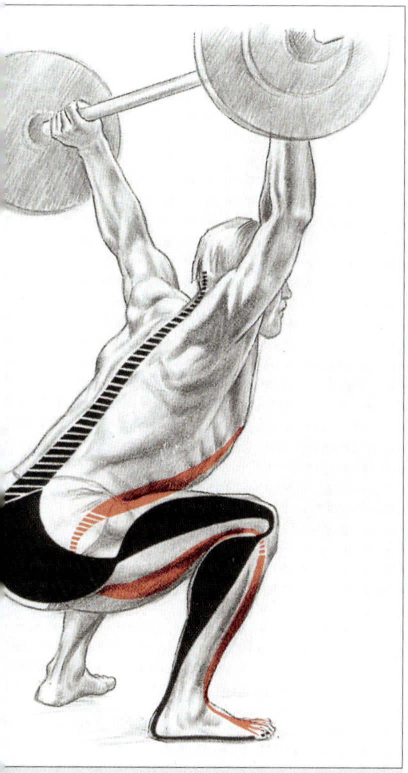

Muscles Fig. 48

- **33** Pectoralis major
- **34** Serratus anterior
- **35** Obliquus externus abdominis
- **39** Trapezius
- **40** Supra- et infraspinatus
- **41** Rhomboideus major
- **42** Latissimus dorsi
- **43** Fascia thoracolumbalis
- **44** Teres major
- **45** Teres minor
- **47** Deltoideus
- **48** Triceps brachii
- **48d** Tendon of Biceps brachii
- **49** Anconeus
- **50** Biceps brachii
- **51** Brachialis
- **52** Coracobrachialis
- **55** Brachioradialis
- **56** Extensor carpi radialis longus
- **57** Extensor carpi radialis brevis
- **58** Extensor carpi ulnaris
- **59** Flexor carpi ulnaris
- **60** Extensor digitorum
- **67** Extensor pollicis brevis
- **68** Abductor pollicis longus
- **78** Gluteus maximus
- **79** Gluteus medius
- **86** Tensor fasciae latae
- **87** Tractus iliotibialis
- **91a** Rectus femoris
- **91b** Vastus lateralis
- **91d** Vastus intermedius
- **94a** Biceps femoris, caput longum
- **94b** Biceps femoris, caput breve
- **99** Gastrocnemius
- **100** Soleus
- **101** Tendo calcaneus
- **102** Tibialis anterior
- **103** Extensor digitorum longus
- **107** Fibularis longus
- **108** Fibularis brevis

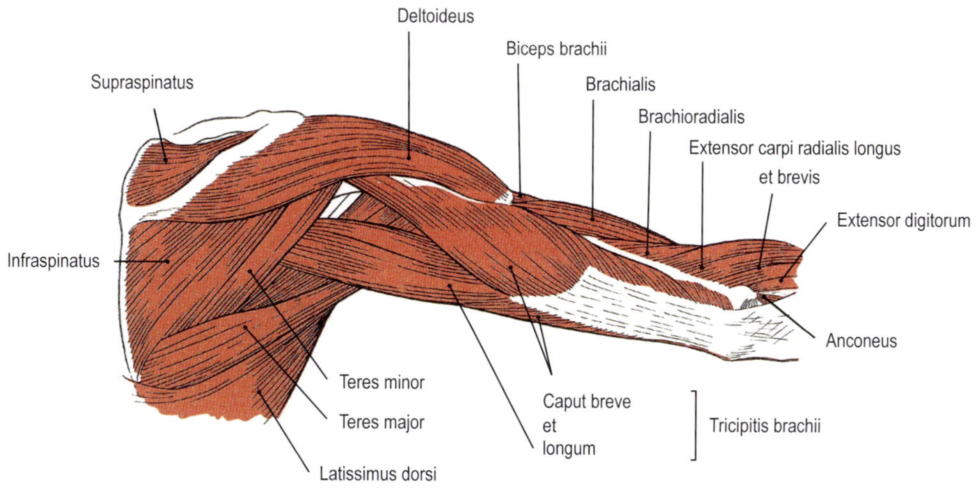

Fig. 49 Shoulder joint and muscles of the upper arm.
In the muscle-sling illustration (fig. 48) only the proportion of the dynamic work, namely the muscles responsible for straightening up the body with their auxillary muscles, is deliberately shown, whereas the proportion of the motor system responsible for statics is only sketched in as it will be considered in greater detail in the following chapters.

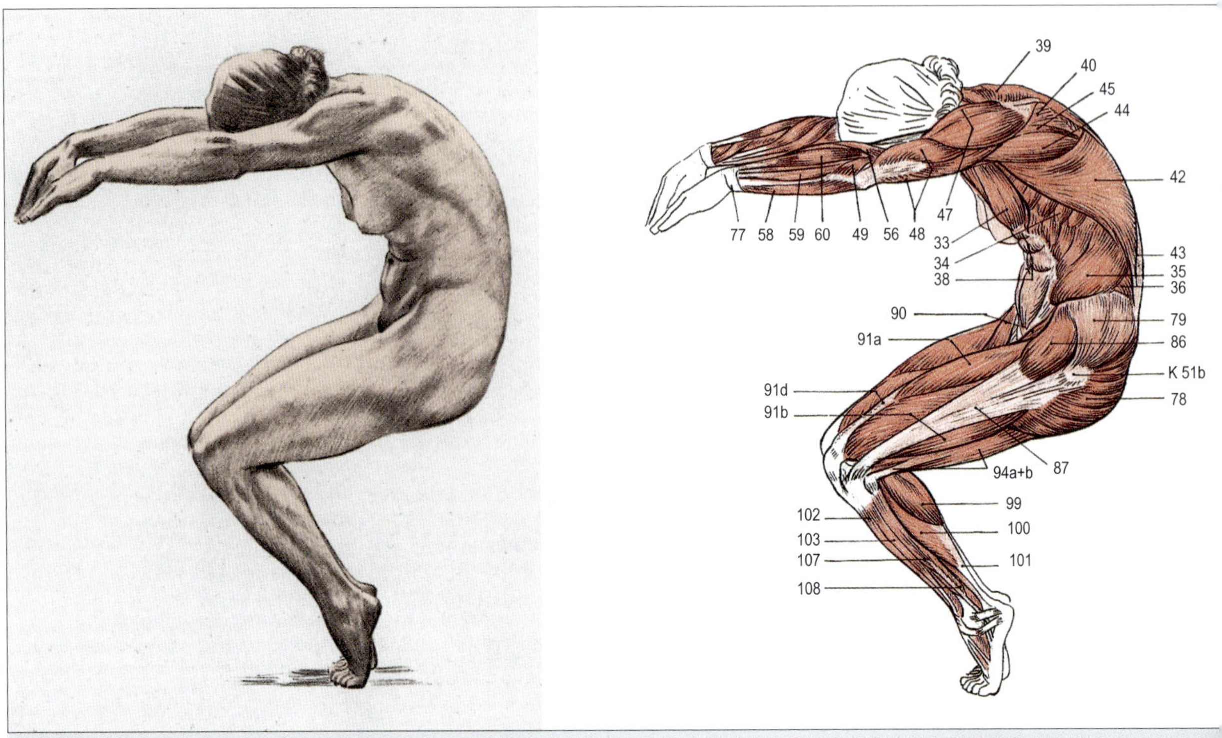

Fig. 50 Inhibitory or braking function of the extensor sling.

Inhibitory and braking function of the extensor sling

The extensor sling shown – this should be mentioned in conclusion – does not only function as an extensor but, by means of its tension, also as a **brake on the movement** by holding the body in a slight knee flexion and on tip-toe (fig. 50). When the trunk is inclined far backwards the centre of gravity is clearly shifted posteriorly to the axis of the knee joint so that gravity exerts a flexing effect.

"The greater the distance between the axis of the centre of gravity and the axis of the knee joint, the greater the torque moment of gravity, the greater the tension of the quadriceps femoris must be in order to maintain the system in equilibrium. Without this muscle it is not possible to flex the knee from a standing position. The distance between the axis of the centre of gravity and the axis of the knee is greatest when the thigh is positioned horizontally. When the muscle contracts in this position it has to overcome gravity by means of its increased tension. This description makes clear the main effect of the extensors and at the same helps us to understand the fact that the extensors which work against gravity must be stronger than the flexors." (Benninghoff, 1931).

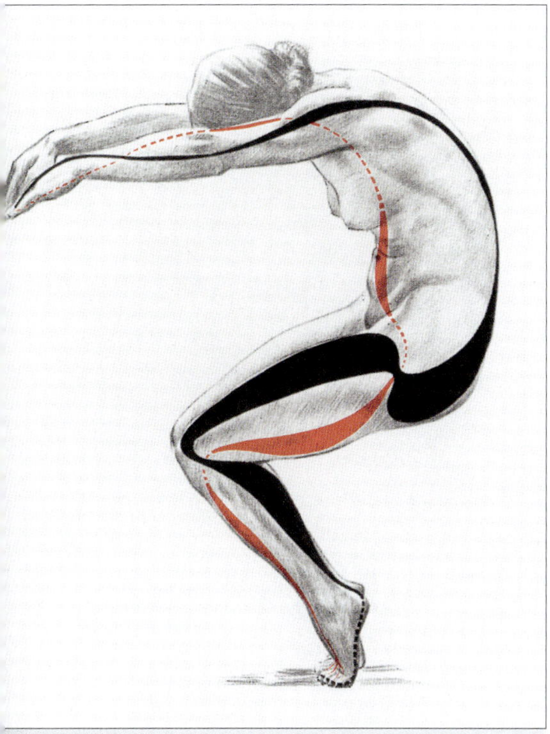

Muscles Fig. 50

- **33** Pectoralis major
- **34** Serratus anterior
- **35** Obliquus externus abdominis
- **36** Obliquus internus abdominis
- **38** Rectus abdominis
- **39** Trapezius
- **40** Supra- et infraspinatus
- **42** Latissimus dorsi
- **43** Fascia thoracolumbalis
- **44** Teres major
- **45** Teres minor
- **47** Deltoideus
- **48** Triceps brachii
- **49** Anconeus
- **56** Extensor carpi radialis longus
- **58** Extensor carpi ulnaris
- **59** Flexor carpi ulnaris
- **60** Extensor digitorum
- **77** Ligg. carpometacarpalia
- **78** Gluteus maximus
- **79** Gluteus medius
- **86** Tensor fasciae latae
- **87** Tractus iliotibialis
- **90** Sartorius
- **91a** Rectus femoris
- **91b** Vastus lateralis
- **91d** Vastus intermedius
- **94a** Biceps femoris, caput longum
- **94b** Biceps femoris, caput breve
- **99** Gastrocnemius
- **100** Soleus
- **101** Tendo calcaneus
- **102** Tibialis anterior
- **103** Extensor digitorum longus
- **107** Fibularis longus
- **108** Fibularis brevis

- **K51b** Trochanter major

This "brake power" plays an important part in many sequences of movements in sport. This can be seen when the athlete lands after a jump, in hand- and volleyball, in the long jump and triple jump, in ski-jumping and in the frequently complicated and risky dismounting from gymnastic equipment. Here a "safe landing" on snow or on the floor of the gymnasium has a crucial influence on the points awarded for the jump or the gymnastic exercise by the jury.

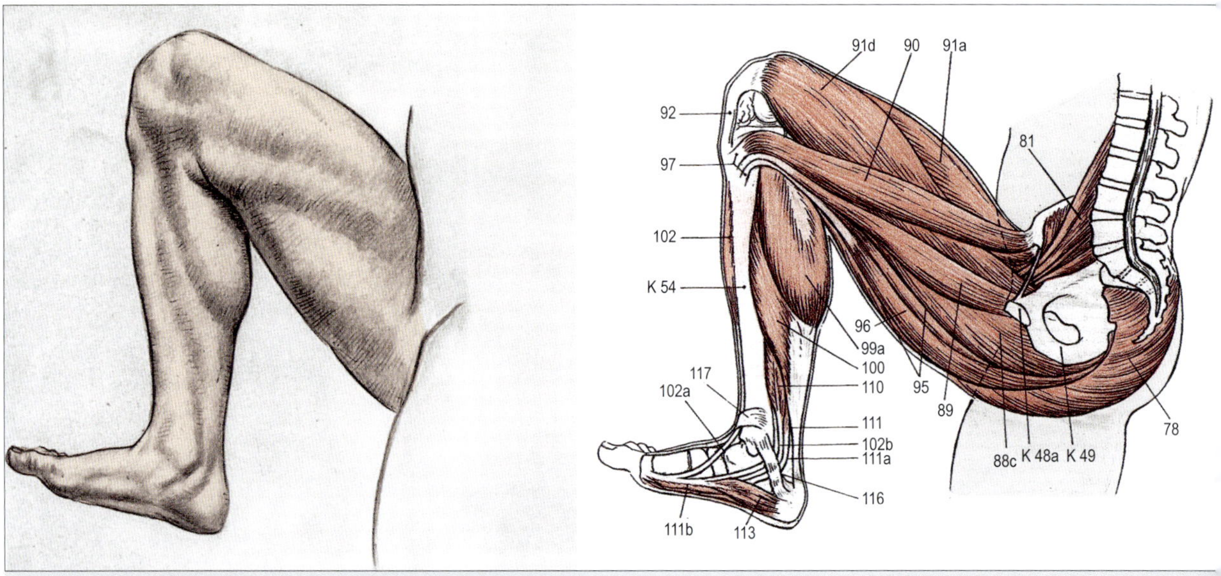

Fig. 51 Basic movement to illustrate the flexor sling in the lower extremity.

2.3 Flexor slings of the lower extremity

Basic movements

The next basic movement (fig. 51) involves a sling which is required, among other things, to lift or to jerk the leg upwards. **The most important muscle for this kind of sequence of movements is the iliopsoas** (fig. 52).

The iliopsoas consists of the **psoas major** which originates from the bodies of the 12th thoracic and the 1st–4th lumbar vertebrae, as well as from the transversal processes of all the lumbar vertebrae, and of the **iliacus,** which originates from the internal surface of the os ilium. The small and slender **psoas minor** can be seen in only 30 % of cases. The common final tendon of the two muscles just mentioned runs underneath the inguinal ligament and is inserted at the lesser trochanter (trochanter minor) of the femur. Thus the iliopsoas lies anteriorly and underneath the pivot of the hip joint.

Because of the fact that the origin of **the iliopsoas** extends a long way cranially along the spine – the higher the origin of a muscle, the greater the lifting height –this muscle **is one of the most important muscles which extend over several joints of the body.** When it is contracted, it is not only the most powerful flexor of the free leg (as opposed to the weight-bearing leg) at the hip joint, but it also moves the lumbar spine and the pelvis at the weight-bearing leg forwards and downwards around a transversal axis running through the hip joints, as can be seen, for example, when raising the

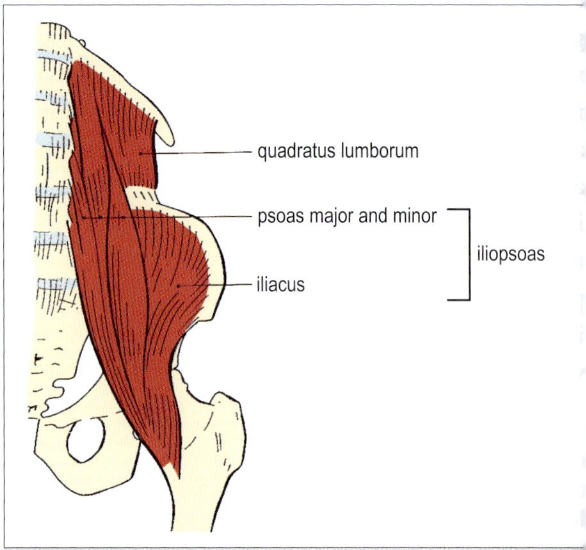

Fig. 52 Internal hip/pelvic muscles

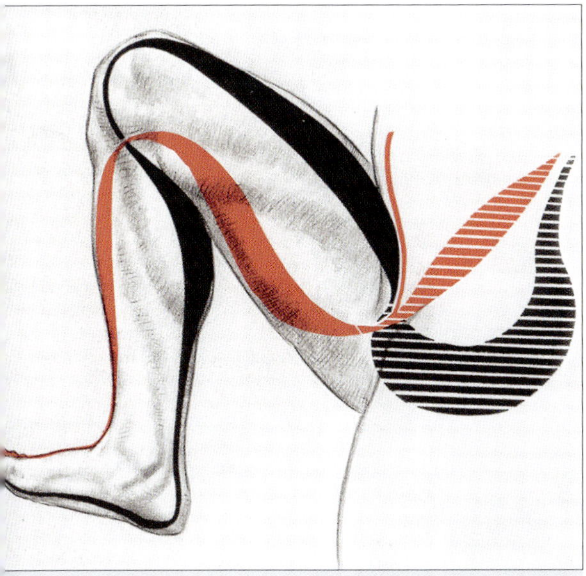

Muscles Fig. 51

78 Gluteus maximus
81 Iliopsoas
88c Adductor magnus
89 Gracilis
90 Sartorius
91a Rectus femoris
91d Vastus intermedius
92 Lig. patellae
95 Semimembranosus
96 Semitendinosus
97 Pes anserinus
99a Gastrocnemius, caput mediale
100 Soleus
102 Tibialis anterior
102a Tendo m. tibialis anterioris
102b Tendo m. flexoris digitorum longi
110 Flexor digitorum longus
111 Flexor hallucis longus
111a Tendo m. flexoris hallucis longi
111b Flexor hallucis brevis
113 Abductor hallucis
116 Retinaculum musculorum extensorum superius
117 Retinaculum musculorum extensorum inferius

K48a Symphysis pubica
K49 Os ischii
K54 Tibia

upper part of the body from a supine position. **It is the muscle which is most utilized for walking, climbing stairs, running and jumping,** because it moves, from a state of extension, the weight-bearing leg with great power from a backward position forwards, upwards and outwards.

In this context we would like to draw attention to the **interplay between the iliopsoas and the gluteus maximus,** which is very impressive in rowing (fig. 41 and 42) or in climbing stairs, the most strenuous physical activity in everyday life, and to the **coordination of the iliopsoas and the abdominal muscles.** The latter are often neglected in power training. It can sometimes be observed that athletes adopt a "hollow-back" position during power training which puts extra stress on the intervertebral discs, but which can be avoided by well-developed abdominal muscles.

! For this reason one should begin with the specific strengthening of the straight and transverse abdominal muscles (rectus and obliquus abdominis), for which sit-ups are suitable, with **flexed legs** and possibly with increasing resistance (with weighted vests), or raising the **flexed or extended legs** above the horizontal position when hanging on to wall bars, before the iliopsoas becomes involved in the power training.

The course of the slings (fig. 51) is very similar to that of the slings described so far, with the difference that in this case the portion of the flexors dominates because of their powerful contraction. The iliopsoas is illustrated in a strictly schematic manner. The (red) flexor sling consists of the following muscles:

- the **flexors of the thigh at the hip joint:** the iliopsoas, the rectus femoris, the tensor fasciae latae, the sartorius, the gluteus minimus as well as the adductor longus and brevis muscles;
- the **flexors of the lower leg at the knee joint:** the semimembranosus, the semitendinosus, the long and short heads of the biceps femoris; and
- the **dorsal extensors at the upper ankle joint:** the tibialis anterior, the extensor hallucis longus as well as the extensor digitorum longus.

The following sequences of movements were chosen to demonstrate the flexor sling which, despite the variety of the sport disciplines discussed, remains largely constant in its course.

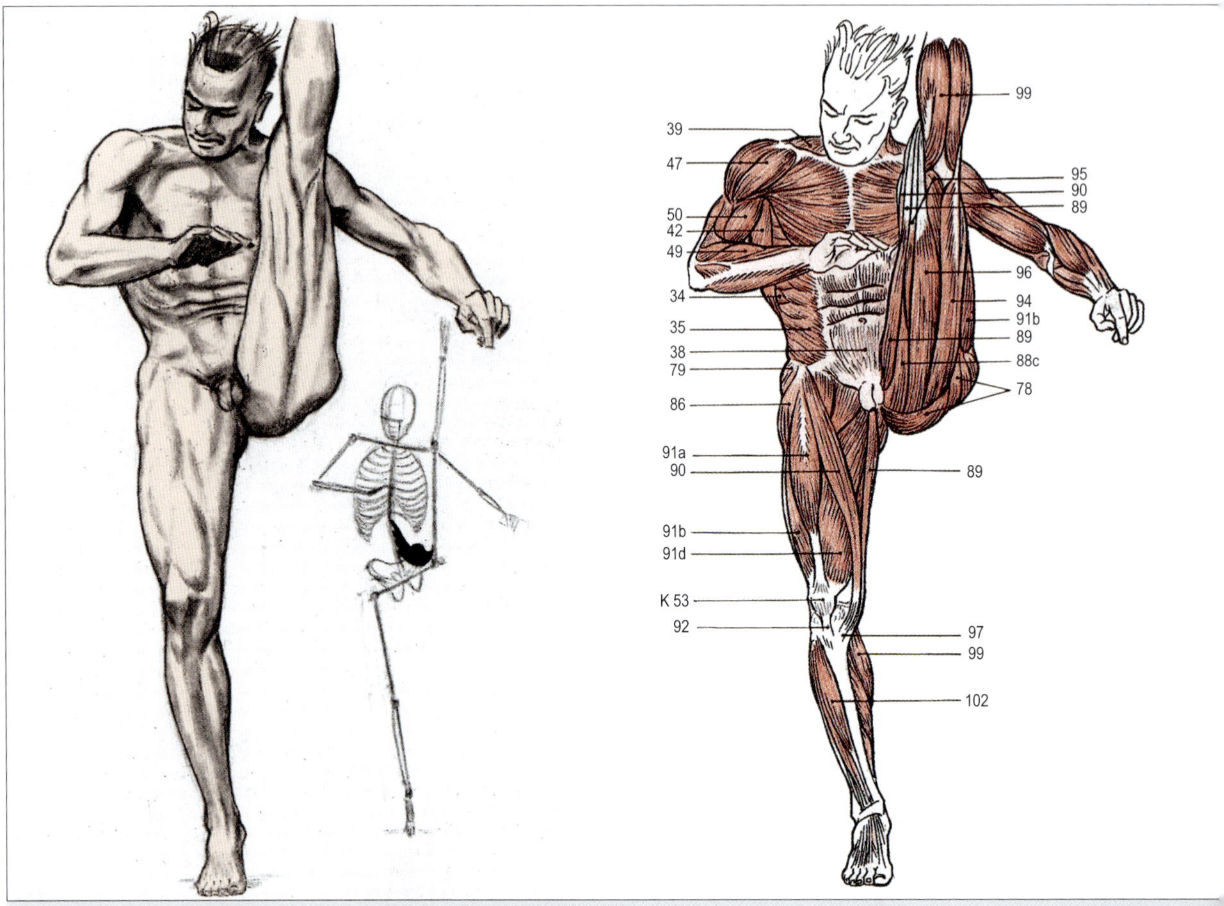

Fig. 53 Sudden lifting of the left leg. The only muscles labelled are those on the posterior side of the left lower extremitiy in order to make it possible for the reader to label the rest of the muscles her-/himself.

Sudden and brisk lifting of the leg

Fig. 53 illustrates a very powerful, explosive sudden lifting of the left leg, in which the thigh almost touches the abdomen. A skeleton has been added to the naturalistic picture in order to give an overview of the **iliopsoas** in its spatial extension Fig. 52. As has already been indicated above, it is only this muscle which is capable of lifting the leg to such a height. In addition, a backwards tilting of the pelvis is necessary, which can be seen in the compressed folds of skin above the navel and the pronounced curvature of the lumbar spine (as an inevitable consequence of the tilting of the pelvis). This process is performed by the gluteus maximus bilaterally, and by the obliquus externus abdominis in cooperation with the left internal obliquus abdominis. Such a pronounced backward tilting of the pelvis inevitably exposes the body to the risk of losing its equilibrium and of falling backwards, which is counteracted by lifting the arms forwards and to the sides. In addition the muscles of the right thigh tend to pull the pelvis forward or, in other words, to prevent an excessive backward tilting, which is visible in the powerfully contracted quadriceps femoris and tensor fasciae latae.

In this context it is important to mention **the gluteus medius and minimus muscles.** These two muscles, which originate at the outer surface of the os ilium and are inserted at the trochanter major of the femur, abduct the leg at the hip joint or incline the pelvis forward (when the thigh is fixated)

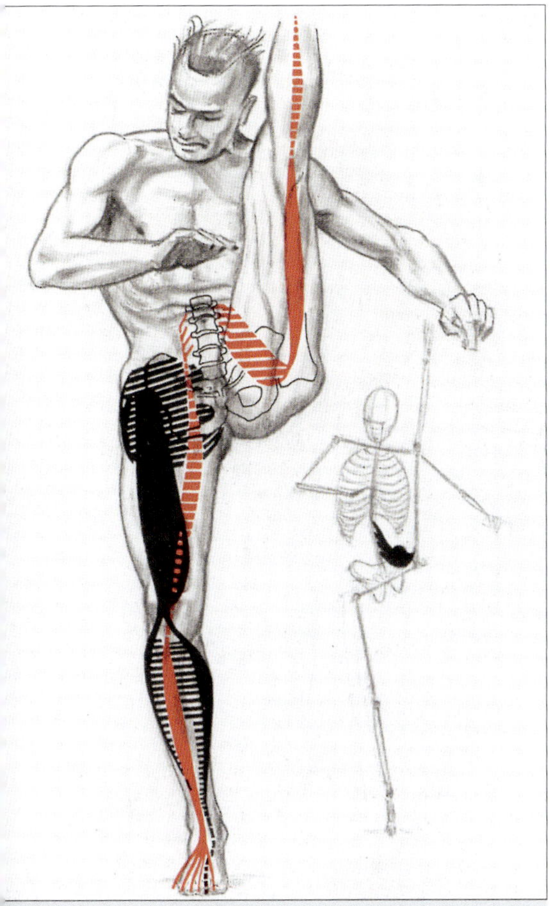

Muscles Fig. 53

34 Serratus anterior
35 Obliquus externus abdominis
38 Rectus abdominis
39 Trapezius
42 Latissimus dorsi
47 Deltoideus
49 Anconeus
50 Biceps brachii
78 Gluteus maximus
79 Gluteus medius
86 Tensor fasciae latae
88c Adductor magnus
89 Gracilis
90 Sartorius
91a Rectus femoris
91b Vastus lateralis
91d Vastus intermedius
92 Lig. patellae
94 Biceps femoris
95 Semimembranosus
96 Semitendinosus
97 Pes anserinus
99 Gastrocnemius
102 Tibialis anterior

K53 Patella

and thereby raise the other (contralateral) half of the pelvis, so that, for example, by contracting the gluteus medius and minimus muscles on the side of the weight-bearing leg, the non-weight-bearing (free) leg can be swung forward more easily.

If only one leg – as in our illustration – has contact with the ground, **both muscles stabilize the position of the pelvis.** They prevent a sideward tilting of the upper body. Tables 11 and 12 provide information about the functioning of the adductors of the thigh at the hip joint and of their antagonists, the abductors of the thigh at the hip joint.

Table 11: Work potential of the adductors of the thigh at the hip joint.

	kg/m
Iliopsoas	5.8
Pectineus	3.7
Adductor brevis	9.0
Adductor longus	12.2
Adductor magnus	28.0
Gracilis	2.9
Semimembranosus	8.4
Semitendinosus	3.9
Biceps femoris, long head	5.5
Gluteus maximus	12.5
Gastrocnemius	3.2
Obturatorius externus	3.7
Quadratus femoris	2.2
All adductors	99.4

Table 12: Work potential of the abductors of the thigh at the hip joint.

	kg/m
Rectus femoris	12.3
Tensor fasciae latae	18.5
Sartorius	1.9
Gluteus maximus, part radiating to the fascia lata	14.0
Gluteus medius	19.0
Gluteus minimus	9.2
Piriformis	1.8
All abductors	76.7

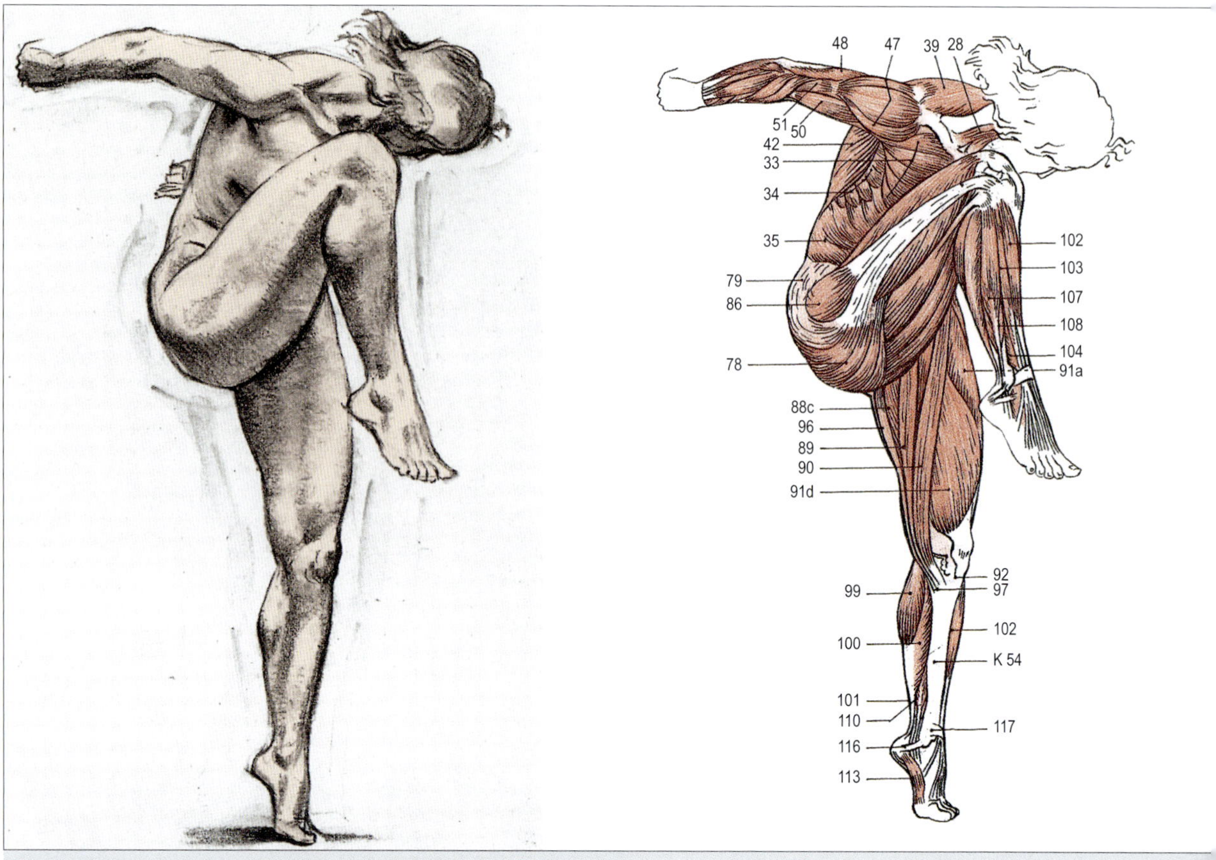

Fig. 54 Flexor sling in the area of the lower extremity in a ballet dancer.

Ballet dancer

In the case of the ballet dancer (fig. 54), the flexor sling (see sling illustration) is similar to what was already discussed in the basic movement (fig. 55). However it should be noted that the course of the sling with extreme **plantar flexion** of the right foot at the upper ankle joint peters out primarily in the calf muscles, the gastrocnemius and the soleus, which are not prominently shown in the illustration. The sequence of movements in ballet, which belongs to the technical and compositional sport disciplines, shows what great demands are put on the active mobility **(flexibility)** of the spine, the shoulders, the elbows, the hands, the hips, the knees, the ankle and toe joints as is also the case in standard ballroom dancing (waltz, tango, slow foxtrot, quickstep) and in the Latin American dances (samba, cha cha cha, rumba and paso doble). In order to be able to adopt the basic ballet position, it is an anatomical condition that the leg is outwardly rotated at an angle of 60–70° at the hip joint.

The great mobility necessary for this movement is often restricted by insufficient elasticity of the calf muscles, the hip flexors, the quadriceps femoris or the dorsal extensors and the plantar flexors of the upper ankle joint. For this reason – taking into consideration and exploiting individual characteristics – **relaxation and stretching** (especially of asymmetrically developed muscles) are of great practical importance. To achieve this one can make use of both active as well as passive stretching, the latter by means of external force. It is the contraction-relaxation-stretching method – also known as PNF-method (proprioceptive neuromuscular facilitation) – which has proved to

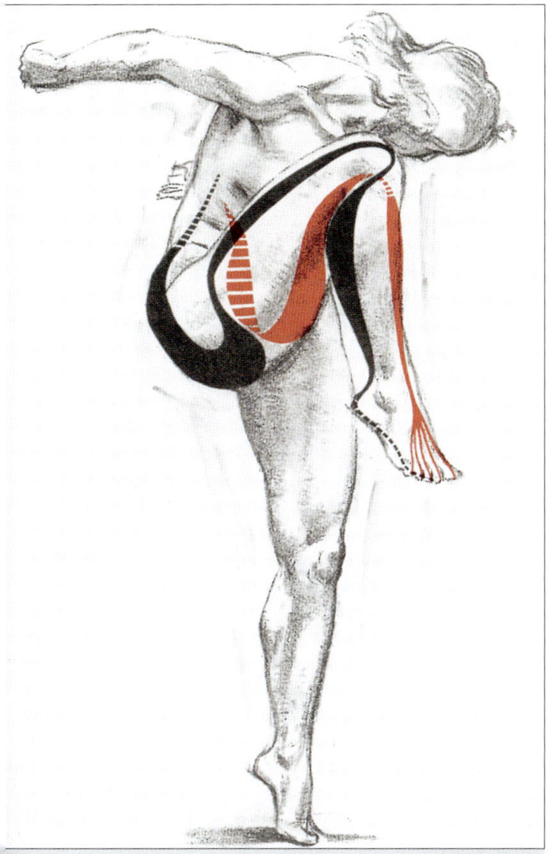

Muscles Fig. 54

28 Sternocleidomastoideus
33 Pectoralis major
34 Serratus anterior
35 Obliquus externus abdominis
39 Trapezius
42 Latissimus dorsi
47 Deltoideus
48 Triceps brachii
50 Biceps brachii
51 Brachialis
78 Gluteus maximus
79 Gluteus medius
86 Tensor fasciae latae
88c Adductor magnus
89 Gracilis
90 Sartorius
91a Rectus femoris
91d Vastus intermedius
92 Lig. patellae
96 Semitendinosus
97 Pes anserinus
99 Gastrocnemius
100 Soleus
101 Tendo calcaneus
102 Tibialis anterior
103 Extensor digitorum longus
104 Extensor digitorum brevis
107 Fibularis longus
108 Fibularis brevis
110 Flexor digitorum longus
113 Abductor hallucis
116 Retinaculum musculorum extensorum superius
117 Retinaculum musculorum extensorum inferius

K54 Tibia

be most effective. It is applied as a series of movements in three phases:

- slow passive stretching of the muscle group which is as relaxed as possible
- static contraction of the stretched muscles and
- further stretching supported by contraction of the antagonistic muscle group.

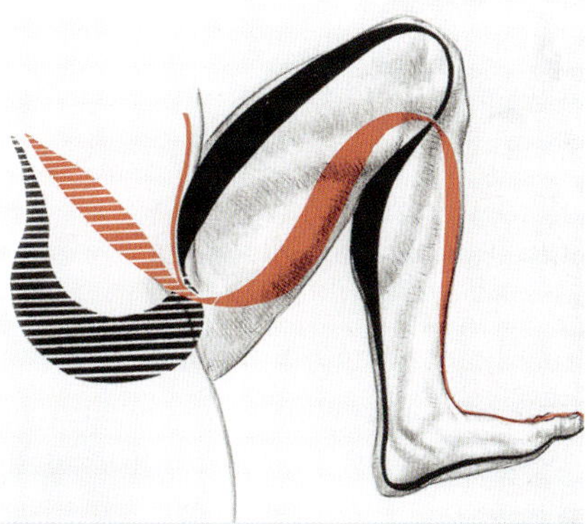

Abb. 55 Compare the course of the muscle slings in the basic movement with the course in the ballet dancer.

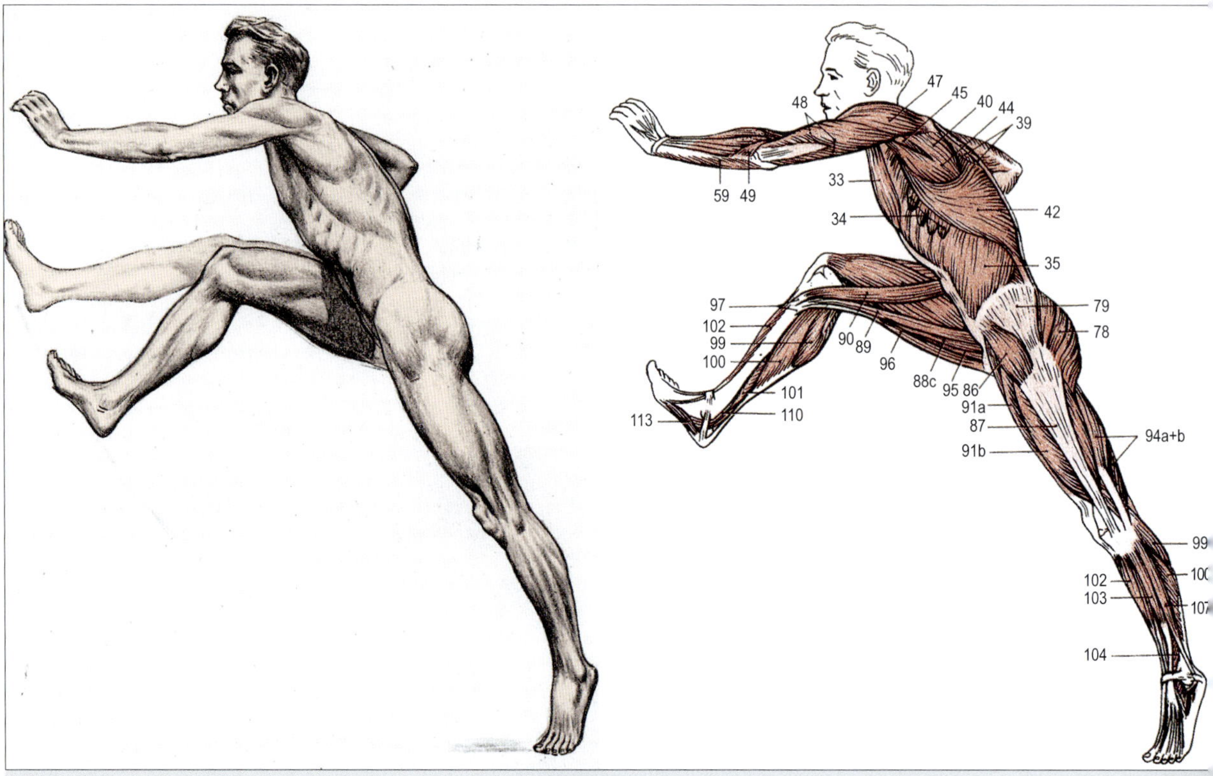

Fig. 56 Flexor and extensor sling over the whole body of a hurdler.

2.4 Flexor and extensor slings in whole-body movements

Hurdler

The movements of the hurdler (fig. 56) are very typical for the activity of the extensor and flexor sling in sequences of movements which involve and control the activity of the hip, knee and ankle joints. This track-and-field discipline demands, in addition to speed and power, distinctive coordinative capabilities for a high degree of active mobility at the hip joint (abduction) and in the lower part of the spine, so that the athlete can jump over the hurdles with an adequate length of stride in the shortest possible time and, after touching down after taking the hurdle, to continue the sprint fluently (without losing speed). The illustration shows the moment of taking the hurdle: the hurdler, who is at an advantage if his upper body and legs are long, takes off from the track by extending his left leg, inclining his upper body far forwards (in order to jump over the hurdle as evenly as possible) and suddenly pulling his right leg upwards and forwards. At the same time the lower leg is catapulted upwards – which is not yet completed in the naturalistic and sling illustrations. Immediately after jumping over the hurdle (whic is 106 cm high and 120 cm wide) the right foot i lowered and touches down on the balls of the foot At the same time the knee joint is extended and th upper body is inclined slightly forwards.

The **participation of the arms** is very noticeabl in the hurdler – which can be clearly seen in th illustrations and which is something we have alread seen when the sprinter starts from a crouching po sition (fig. 57). These **active pendular movement** (ante- and retroversion) **act as a brake on the rotar movements of the body** at the heads of the femu in the hip joint during walking and running. Th left arm begins to swing forwards shortly before th right leg is brought forwards. By comparison, whe we are walking or running slowly and strenuousl uphill, the arms swing only a little, whereas whe we are walking and running downhill the arms hav a wide amplitude and sometimes swing twice a

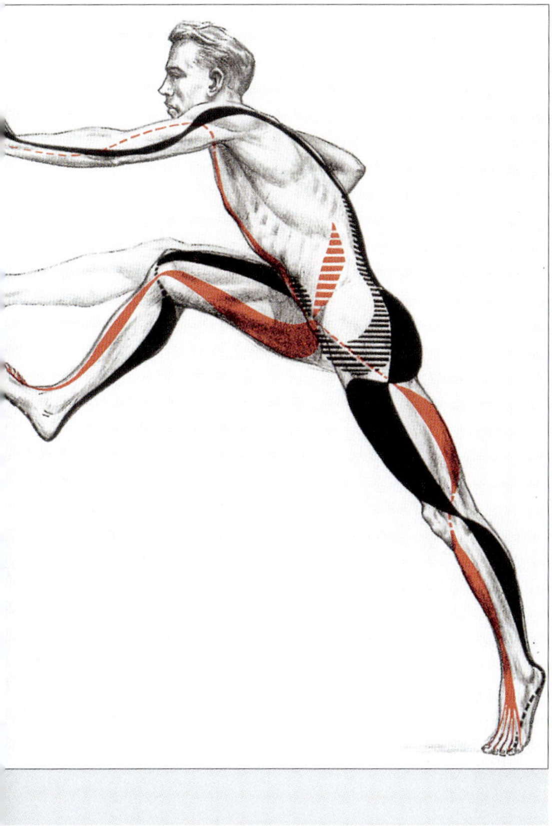

Muscles Fig. 56

33 Pectoralis major
34 Serratus anterior
35 Obliquus externus abdominis
39 Trapezius
40 Supra- et infraspinatus
42 Latissimus dorsi
44 Teres major
45 Teres minor
47 Deltoideus
48 Triceps brachii
49 Anconeus
59 Flexor carpi ulnaris
78 Gluteus maximus
79 Gluteus medius
86 Tensor fasciae latae
87 Tractus iliotibialis
88c Adductor magnus
89 Gracilis
90 Sartorius
91a Rectus femoris
91b Vastus lateralis
94a Biceps femoris, caput longum
94b Biceps femoris, caput breve
95 Semimembranosus
96 Semitendinosus
97 Pes anserinus
99 Gastrocnemius
100 Soleus
101 Tendo calcaneus
102 Tibialis anterior
103 Extensor digitorum longus
104 Extensor digitorum brevis
107 Fibularis longus
110 Flexor digitorum longus
113 Abductor hallucis

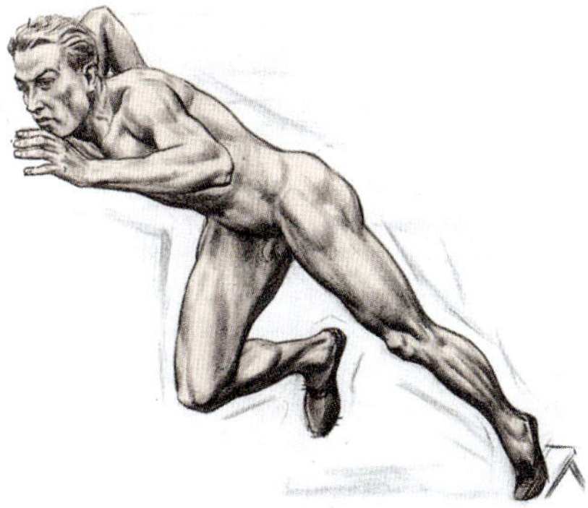

Fig. 57 Sprinter starting from a crouching position (participation of the arms).

fast as the legs because they are accelerated by the contraction of the arm muscles.

In hurdling, in the high jump, in the long jump and in the triple jump – just to mention these disciplines as representative of many others – the centre of gravity of the arms is raised by flinging them upwards (while one foot is still on the ground). The athlete pulls him-/herself upwards towards the new centre of gravity. In landing after jumping – this is especially noticeable in gymnastics and ski jumping – the arms which have been flung upwards serve to maintain the equilibrium of the body.

! This means that the movements of the upper extremities, when we are walking and running, are used for different purposes from those when we are jumping. In the former the movements of the arms alternate on both sides, in the latter they are usual simultaneous.

It can be seen that the hurdler, whose upper body is inclined forwards, does not particularly extend the lower leg at the knee joint on the right. What can be the reason for this? When the thigh is in pronounced flexion at the hip joint and one wants to extend the lower leg from this position (as seen in the illustrations) then one feels that the extension is inhibited by the contracted flexors of the lower leg on the posterior side of the thigh – the biceps femoris and the semimembranosus and semitendinosus muscles – at the knee joint. As soon as the flexion at the hip joint is released, the tension of the flexors of the lower leg recedes, so that nothing stands in the way of a total extension at the knee joint. On the other hand, when the leg is extended at the knee it can only be partially flexed at the hip joint. It is only when the extension is reduced that a greater flexion of the lower extremity at the hip joint becomes possible.

In the sling illustration the extension, which runs from the sole of the left foot over the whole body as far as the ipsilateral hand, can be followed, whereas the sling which consists of several flexors, including the iliopsoas, is shown in the right leg.

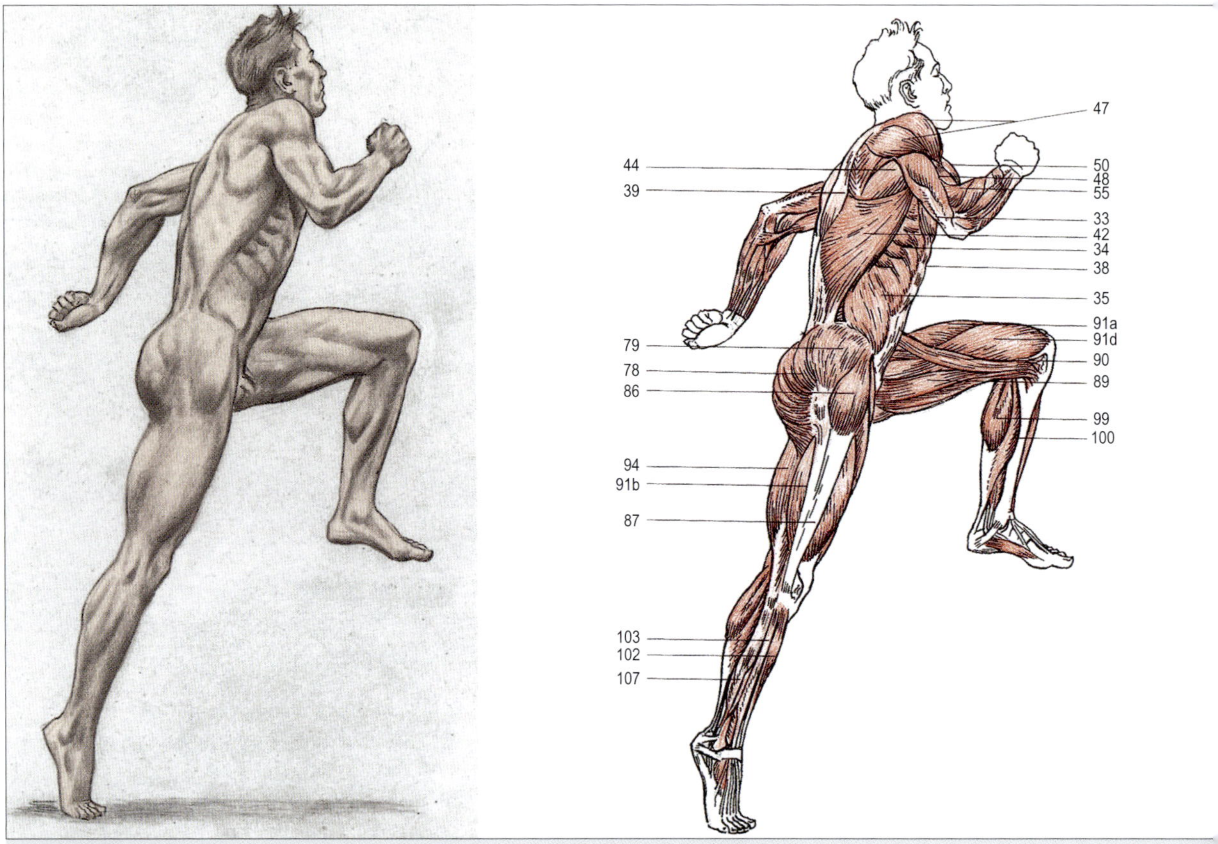

Fig. 58 Flexor and extensor sling over the whole body of a long jumper.

Long jumper

In the long jump (fig. 58) a **cyclic** movement (a powerful 35–45 m long accelerated run-up) and an **acyclic** movement (jump, airborne and landing phase) are combined – as is also the case in the high jumper (fig. 61) and pole vault. The disciplines mentioned have differing airborne phases. For the long jump it is necessary to have high speed and great accuracy in the run-up, an individually optimal step-rhythm, a great flexibility at the hip joint and the lumbar spine (for the landing phase) and a fast and powerful extensor sling.

The **motion study** (Fig. 59) demonstrates in detail that the jumping leg touches the ground first with the heel. During the take-off there is a strong plantar flexion of the foot as well as a maximal extension of the ankle, knee and hip joints by the powerful extensor muscle sling (Fig. 59). The second leg moves forwards and the knee joint is flexed.

In the second part of the **flight phase** of the jump (preparation for landing) the jumper brings both legs as far as possible before the centre of gravity by flexing the upper part of his trunk and his arms forwards. Only this action and the "pen-knife" position guarantee a safe touch-down and a very long jump, perhaps a new world record.

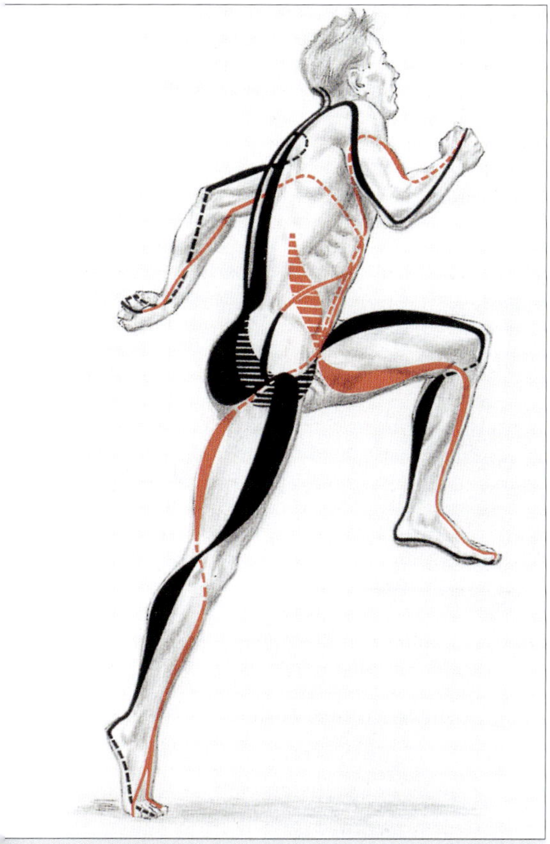

Muscles Fig. 58

- **33** Pectoralis major
- **34** Serratus anterior
- **35** Obliquus externus abdominis
- **38** Rectus abdominis
- **39** Trapezius
- **42** Latissimus dorsi
- **44** Teres major
- **47** Deltoideus
- **48** Triceps brachii
- **50** Biceps brachii
- **55** Brachioradialis
- **78** Gluteus maximus
- **79** Gluteus medius
- **86** Tensor fasciae latae
- **87** Tractus iliotibialis
- **89** Gracilis
- **90** Sartorius
- **91a** Rectus femoris
- **91b** Vastus lateralis
- **91d** Vastus intermedius
- **94** Biceps femoris
- **99** Gastrocnemius
- **100** Soleus
- **102** Tibialis anterior
- **103** Extensor digitorum longus
- **107** Fibularis longus

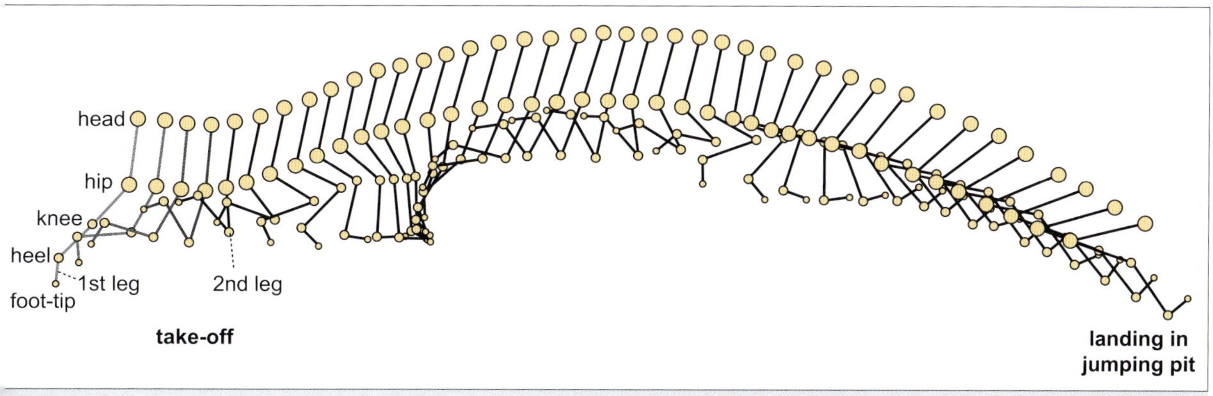

Fig. 59 Slow-motion sketch of an world-class long jump, illustrating the dynamic movements of the whole body during the jump and the abiliy of the athlete to coordinate the single phases in order to transform the kinetic energy, stored during the run-up, from horizontal to vertical energy, necessary to perform the jump.

The world record performances in long jump for men improved from under 6.00 meters in 1866 to 8.35 meters in 1964, but showed surprising periodic fluctuations. For instance, in 1935 **Jesse Owens** achieved a remarkable 8.13 meters, and this long jump record remained unchanged for over 29 years. The question therefore arose of whether the special conditions of the Olympic Summer Games in 1968 in Mexico-City are capable of explaining this change, because an altitude of 2400 meters (or 7.500 ft.) above sea level can cause significant and exceptional increases in performance in track-and-field disciplines.

But who would be able to fulfill these expectations?

Bob Beamon (USA) fulfilled these requirements when he set a new world record of 8.90 m in the long jump, a record which lasted for 23 years.

In 1991 Powel (USA) set a new world record in Tokyo with a jump of 8.95 m. Beamon was able to convert his high starting speed and jumping power by applying his technical movement skills into a long-jump distance, which at that time was hardly considered possible. The author of this book could witness this from a close range in his capacity as on-call physician in the stadium: Beamon made use of his physical characteristics (height 1.91 m, weight 70 kg, favourable leverage due to his longer calf muscles) and the lower air resistance (which makes it possible to sprint quickly) and a reliable tail wind (of 1.99 m/s). The moment of the explosive start of the jump, up to the point where the athlete would have attained maximum start-up speed, is shown in fig. 60.

Beamon's fantastic performance, which electrified everyone who witnessed it, ranks to this day as one of the most remarkable athletic feats of all time. Surprisingly it took longer than 5 minutes to announce the official result, because the range of the specially installed semi-automatic recording unit turned out to be too narrow. The news that he had jumped 8.90 meters did not seem to affect him at all.

When he was told that he had jumped 29 ft. 2½ inches he fell to the ground as if struck by lightening. He inexplicably lost control over the leg muscles for more than 50 seconds and was unable to move voluntarily. We had witnessed a so-called **"cataplectic attack"**, an unusual reaction to happy (or sad) emotion, manifested by a sudden loss of muscle tone. Beamon was undoubtedly surprised himself because his best previous jump had been about half a meter less. His record stimulated research in several disciplines, such as sports science

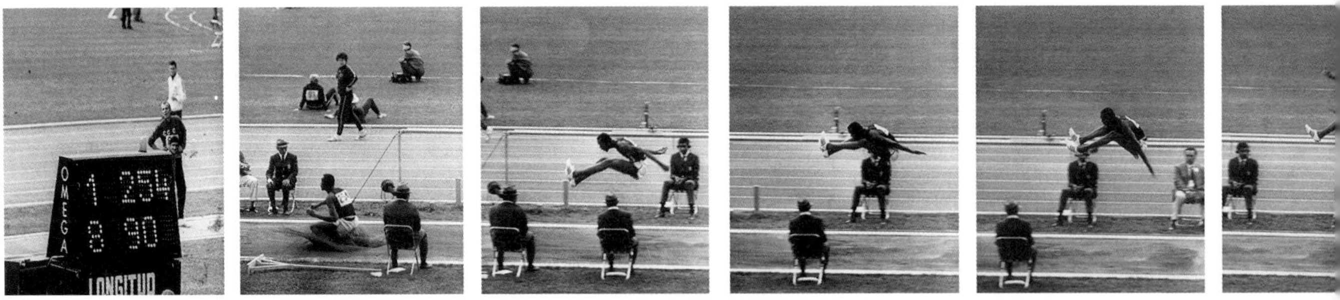

Fig. 60 Beamon's historic long jump. Look from the right to the left at the 12 typical moments of his jump.

and biomechanical and functional anatomy and resulted in increased knowledge of the long and high jump.

In order to be able to jump with power forwards and upwards, the **running speed must be reduced** (from about 9.35 m/s to 8.05 m/s) at the moment when the almost completely extended jumping leg touches down on the track. Immediately after this there is, through the **excentric** work of the **extensor sling,** a further acceleration of the centre of gravity of the body until the jumper's body is completely extended. The **speed increases once more** (from 8.05 m/s to 8.36 m/s). Thus the initial phase of the jump can be subdivided into **a braking and an acceleration phase.** In order to master both of these phases, great power is required (from the beginning to the end of the take-off), and the impulse during the take-off is increased by the swinging movements of the arms.

The landing of the long jumper in the pit is secured mainly by the **flexor sling,** which has to perform a very pronounced flexion at the hip joint, and by the **abdominal muscles.** The extraordinary physical conditions of Bob Beamon already mentioned illustrate clearly some phases of this fantastic jump. The current research results on the functioning of the extensor sling during take-off – the registered power comes to 4950–5900 N – indicate that in the long jump about 60 % – in the high jump about 70 % – of the jumping capability not only of "concentric" but also and above all of "excentric" work must be done. The faster the pre-extension is, the greater are the power moments which thereby arise and the greater the muscle stretching is as well.

> *"If a muscle is stretched by an external factor ('excentric' work) potential energy will be stored as a result of the influence of this stretching on the consecutive series of elastic components which can be used as additional kinetic energy – on condition that the active contraction phase of the muscle ('concentric' work) comes immediately after the pre-extension. In this way the muscles can do more external work without the chemical energy having to be increased. For this reason the elastic component is crucial for external work to be carried out." (Komi, 1975).*

This knowledge has become an integral part of the power training of jumpers, which takes into account the interchange of excentric and concentric work which must take place at the right moment.

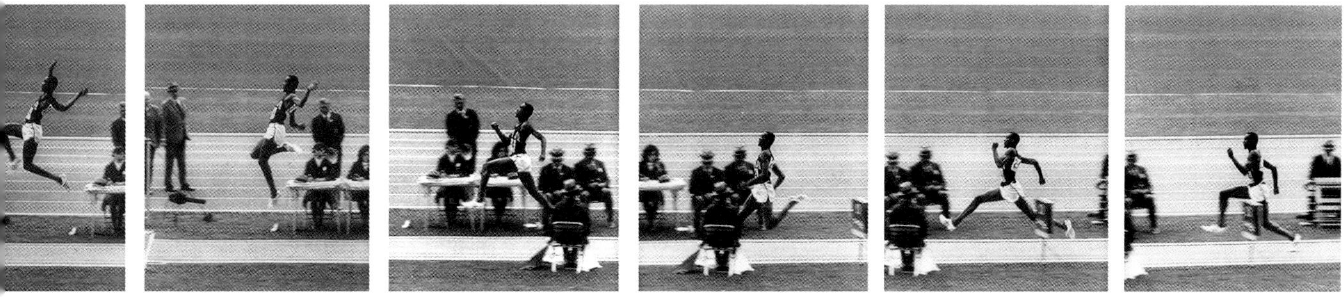

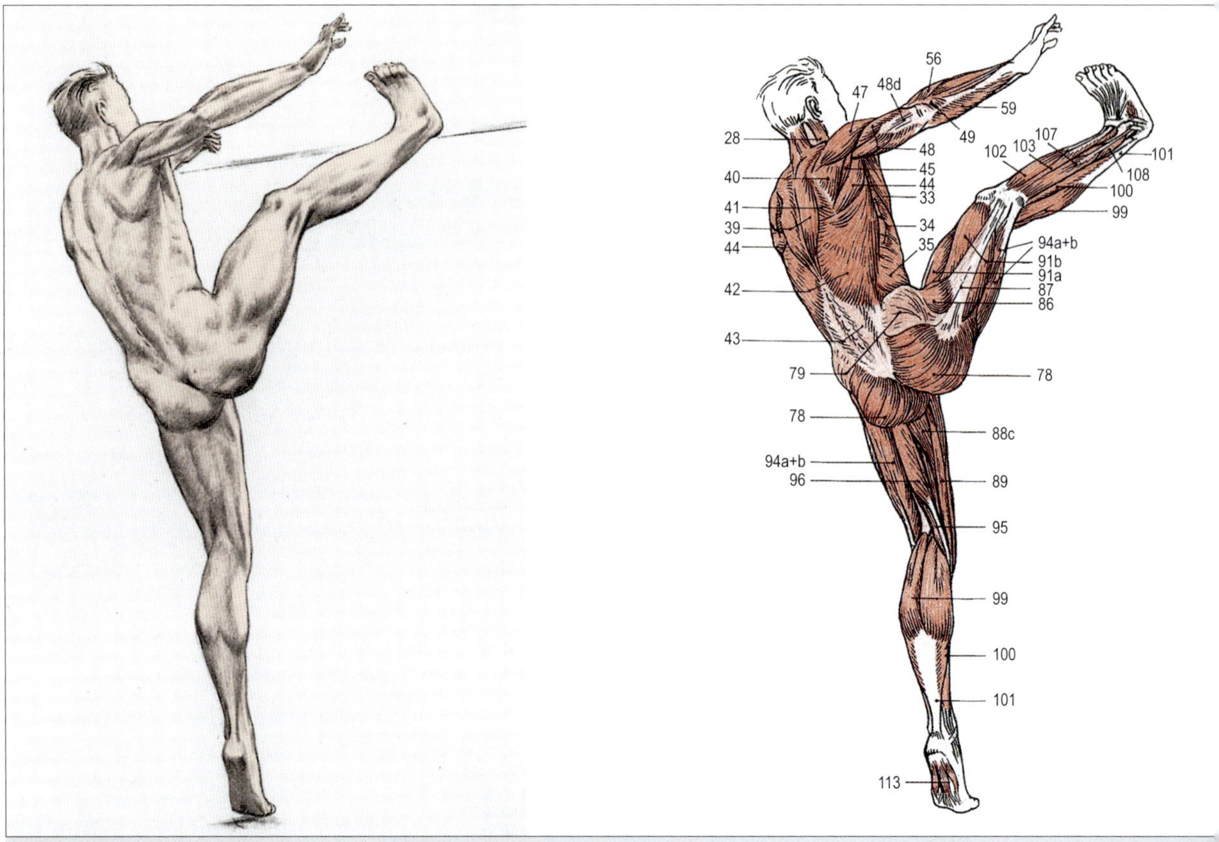

Fig. 61 Flexor and extensor sling over the whole body in a high jumper.

High jumper

In the next sequence of movements, the straddle high jump (fig. 61), which is no longer used and has now been replaced by the Fosbury-flop, there is usually an extreme extension of the left jumping leg and an equally extreme flexion of the free leg at the hip joint. The sequence of movement is characterized by a shortening of the take-off time and, at the same time, an increase in the effectiveness of the take-off. This is achieved by a relatively high run-up speed at the beginning of the take-off (6,5–7,5 m/s) and by a change in the coordination of the movement of the swing elements (almost fully extended jumping leg and arms flung suddenly upwards) at the moment of the take-off. As in the illustration of the long jump, the **rapid sequence of flexion and extension of the jumping or supporting leg** with a simultaneous reduction of the run-up speed in order to brake (slight bending at the knee joint of the jumping leg and thus a pre-extension of the extensors of the lower extremity) becomes clear, and this makes it possible to transfer the kinetic energy achieved in the run-up to the jump power and range.

It should be pointed out once more (see sling illustration) that, with regard to the **stabilization of the lumbo-sacral transition** (fig. 62), it is primarily the **gluteus maximus** together with its antagonist, the **iliopsoas,** which achieves a specific pelvic tilt. The gluteus maximus decreases the angle of pelvic tilt in cooperation with the abdominal muscles, while the iliopsoas increases the angle of pelvic tilt, which causes a stretching of the abdominal muscles.

> *"... because the lower section of the skeletal frame, in which they are clamped, has moved further away from the upper section, the costal-arch. By contracting, the abdominal muscles can lift the tilted pelvis to its initial position. Thus we*

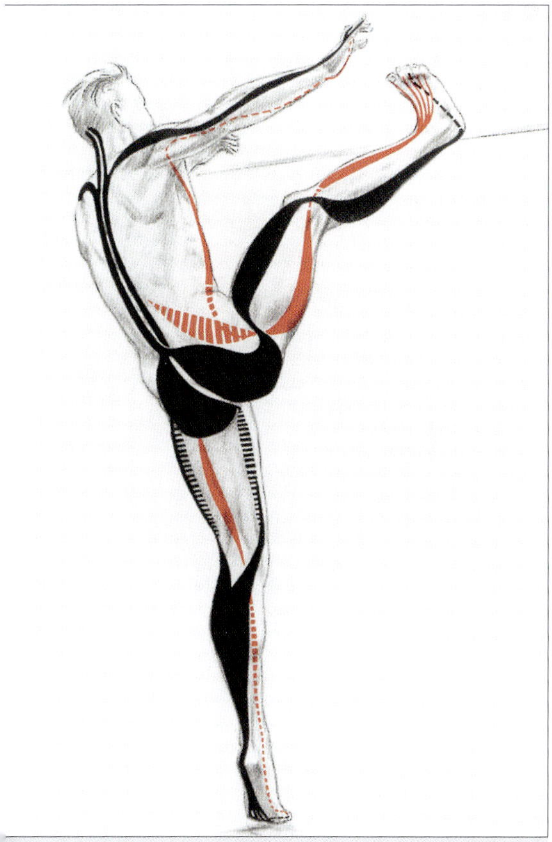

Muscles Fig. 61

28 Sternocleidomastoideus	86 Tensor fasciae latae
33 Pectoralis major	87 Tractus iliotibialis
34 Serratus anterior	88c Adductor magnus
35 Obliquus externus abdominis	89 Gracilis
39 Trapezius	91a Rectus femoris
40 Supra- et infraspinatus	91b Vastus lateralis
41 Rhomboideus major	94a Biceps femoris, caput longum
42 Latissimus dorsi	94b Biceps femoris, caput breve
43 Fascia thoracolumbalis	95 Semimembranosus
44 Teres major	96 Semitendinosus
45 Teres minor	99 Gastrocnemius
47 Deltoideus	100 Soleus
48 Triceps brachii	101 Tendo calcaneus
48d Tendon of triceps brachii	102 Tibialis anterior
49 Anconeus	103 Extensor digitorum longus
56 Extensor carpi radialis longus	107 Fibularis longus
59 Flexor carpi ulnaris	108 Fibularis brevis
78 Gluteus maximus	113 Abductor hallucis
79 Gluteus medius	

can, so to speak, rock the pelvis on the heads of the femur by alternating contraction of the abdominal muscles and the gluteus maximus. Of course the spine is very closely involved in these movements; it must also go along with every change of pelvic tilt, because it is connected to the gluteus maximus via the sacrum, which is inserted into the osseous pelvic bone, and via the fascia thoracolumbalis." (Hoepke, 1971)

This powerful contraction, not only of the gluteus maximus but also of the abdominal muscles and the iliopsoas, should not be overlooked when considering this sequence of movements. Their play and counterplay are supported by a **strong ligamental apparatus,** which prevents extreme changes in pelvic tilt, and which is an important condition for the unimpeded performance of the high jump.

In this connection we should also not forget the activity of the **gluteus medius.** This muscle not only makes coordinated pendular movements of the leg in walking possible, but also prevents the tilting of the pelvis to the side of the free leg when one is standing on one leg.

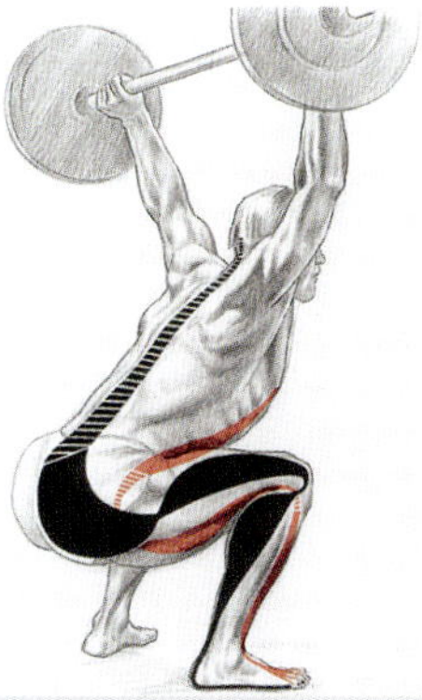

Fig. 62 Sling illustration of the whole body in a weightlifter during the push.

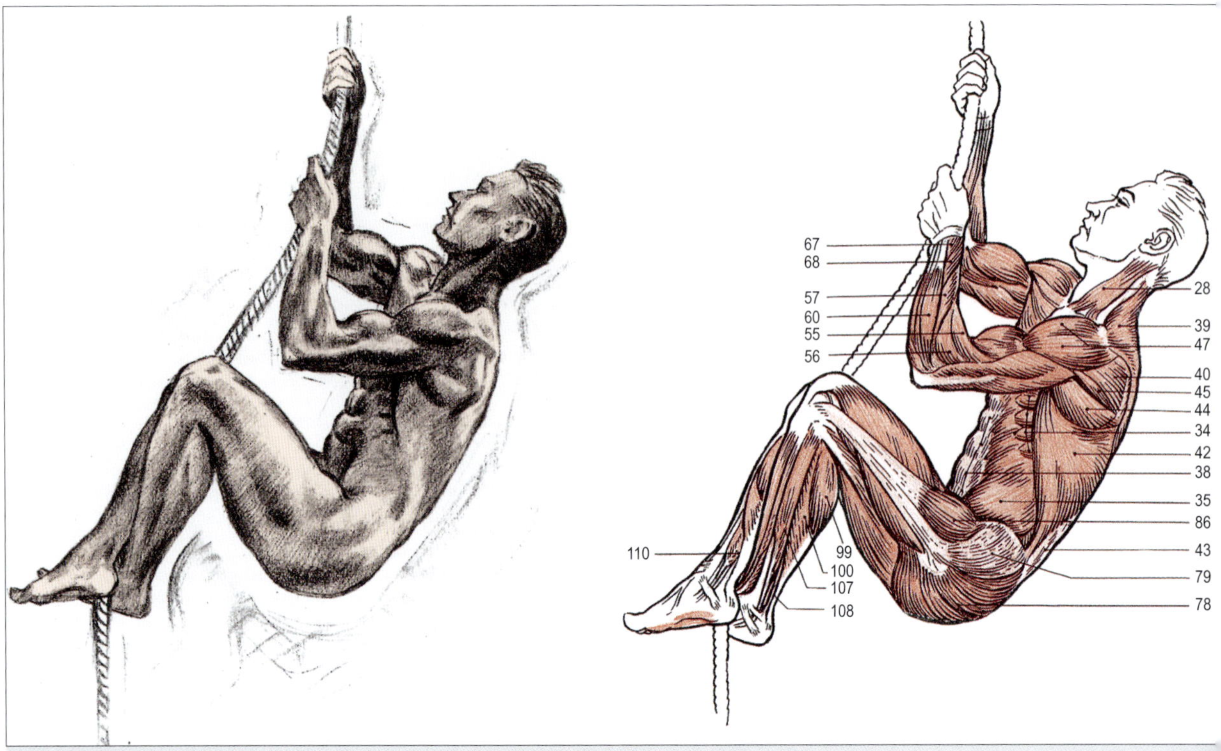

Fig. 63 Flexor and extensor slings over the whole body in a rope climber.

Rope climber

In this last section on the flexor slings (fig. 63), both the flexor and the extensor slings over the whole body of the rope climber show the **interplay between the gluteus maximus and the iliopsoas.** If the latter is contracted, its antagonist is stretched to the same extent at the same time. But if the gluteus maximus with its coarse, strong fibres is contracted, then it pushes the pelvis upwards and forwards, that is, **it raises the trunk against gravity,** which also is important both for climbing stairs.

Wall climber

Virtually the same flexor and extensor muscle slings, combined with the long and short flexors of the hands and fingers, make possible indoor climbing up a wall (fig. 64). They stabilize the trunk so that the centre of gravity, when the athlete is suspended and is climbing, can be brought into an optimal position. This discipline has developed within the last 25 years as a recreational sport for all age groups and as a rehabilitative measure after injury.

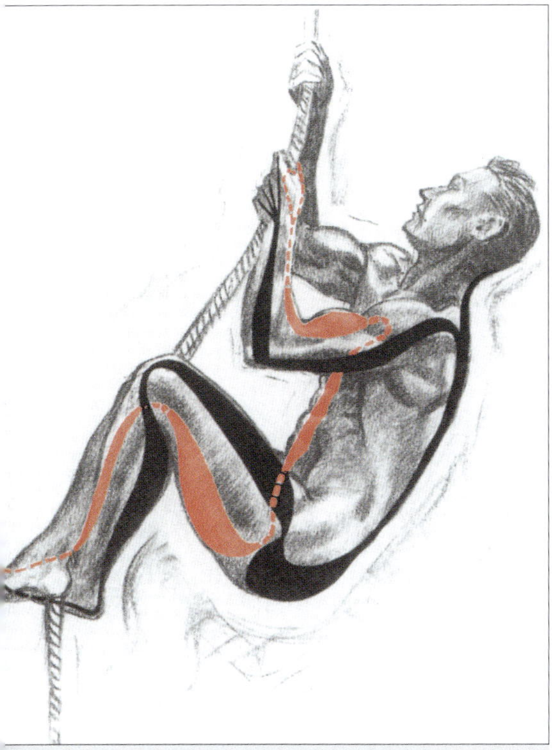

Muscles Fig. 63 and 64

28 Sternocleido-mastoideus
33 Pectoralis major
34 Serratus anterior
35 Obliquus externus abdominis
38 Rectus abdominis
39 Trapezius
40 Supra- et infraspinatus
42 Latissimus dorsi
43 Fascia thoracolumbalis
44 Teres major
45 Teres minor
47 Deltoideus
48 Triceps brachii
50 Biceps brachii
55 Brachioradialis
56 Extensor carpi radialis longus
57 Extensor carpi radialis brevis
58 Extensor carpi radialis brevis
59 Flexor carpi ulnaris
60 Extensor digitorum
67 Extensor pollicis brevis
68 Abductor pollicis longus
78 Gluteus maximus
79 Gluteus medius
86 Tensor fasciae latae
89 Gracilis
90 Sartorius
91 Quadriceps femoris
99 Gastrocnemius
100 Soleus
102 Tibialis anterior
107 Fibularis longus
108 Fibularis brevis
110 Flexor digitorum longus

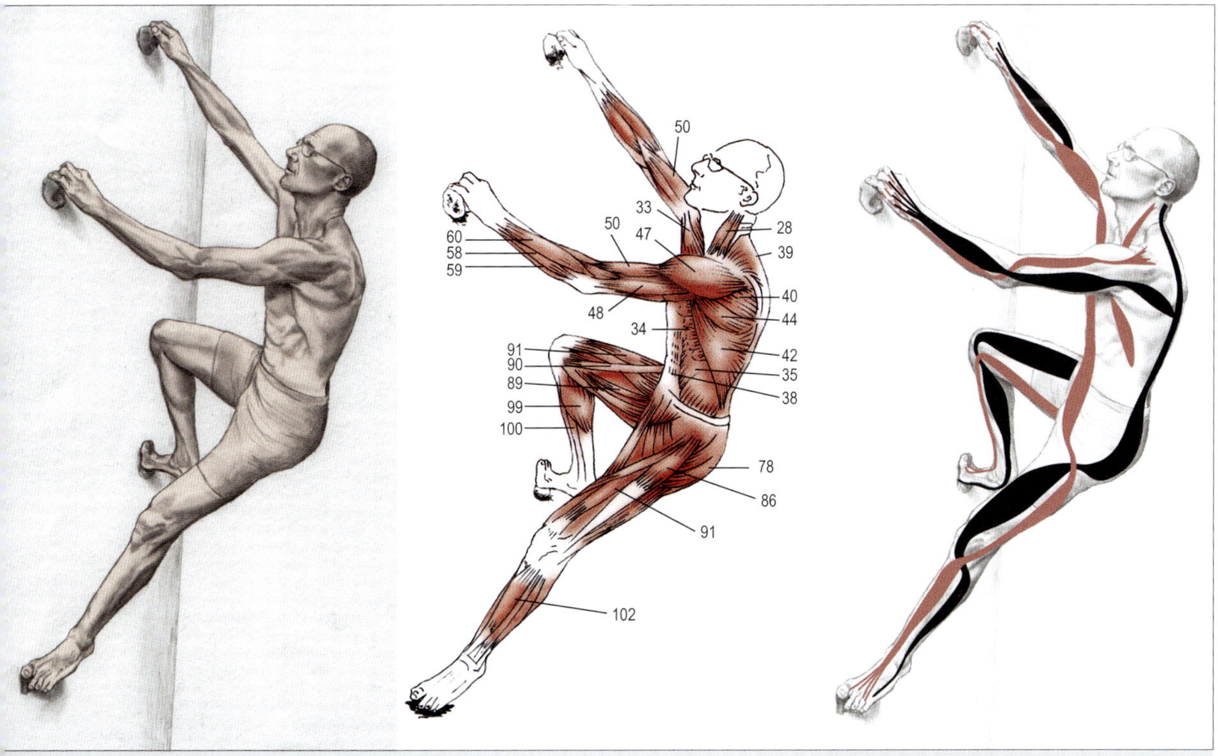

Fig. 64 Wall climber.

Muscles of the trunk and the shoulder girdle in artistic gymnastics

The purely dynamic sequences of movements discussed so far have made the reader familiar with combinations of muscles, which for the most part run from the lower extremities to the upper extremities and include the trunk, which anticipates the movement of the extremities.

The focus of the following sequences of movements in sport is **the trunk with its static function,** secured by a strong "muscle corset" for the maintenance of particular body postures, with its **dynamic function** in absorbing and transferring mild shocks which occur in walking and jumping, with its supportive function for the internal organs of the thoracic and abdominal cavities, and with its complex involvement in partial and whole-body movements. There are muscle slings which are centred mainly on the trunk and which extend upwards from the thorax to the **shoulder girdle and upper arm,** and which are able to lift the body – if the points of origin and insertion are interchanged. This applies, among other things,

- to the latissimus dorsi (fig. 65),
- to the lower strands of the pectoralis major (fig. 66),
- to the pectoralis minor (fig. 67), and
- to the lower strands of the serratus anterior (fig. 68)
- and the rhomboids, as well as the ascending parts of the trapezius (fig. 69).

Because most of their fibres run obliquely upwards, these muscles are generally much more strongly developed than the muscles with fibres which run horizontally or downwards. The former support not only the movements of the free arm at the shoulder joint but also secure the weight of the body and its fixation at the fixated arm (see below).

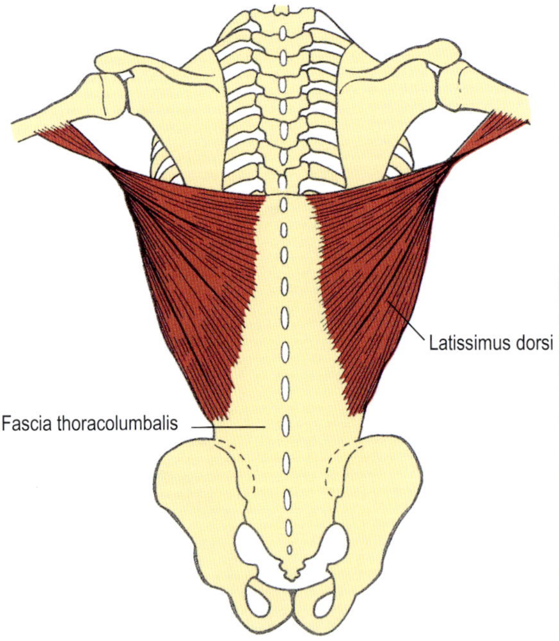

Fig. 65 The broad muscle of the back: latissimus dorsi.

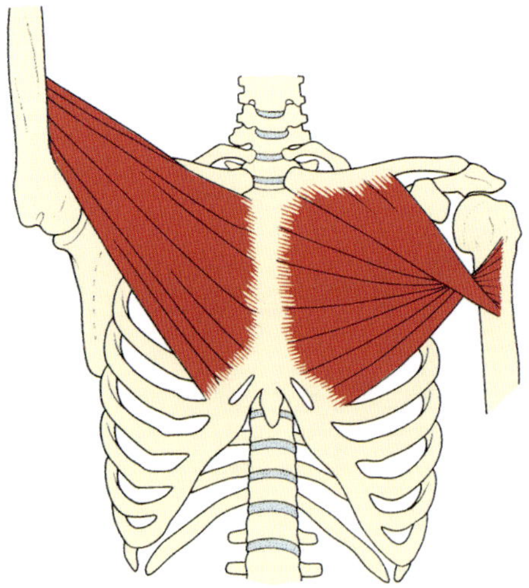

Fig. 66 Pectoralis major: Crossing-over of the fibre strands before the point of insertion at rest and the unwinding of the fibres when the arm is raised.

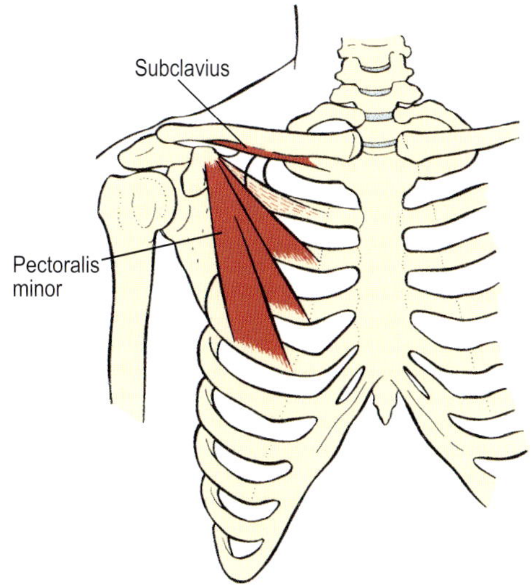

Fig. 67 The anterior muscles of the shoulder girdle: Pectoralis minor and subclavius.

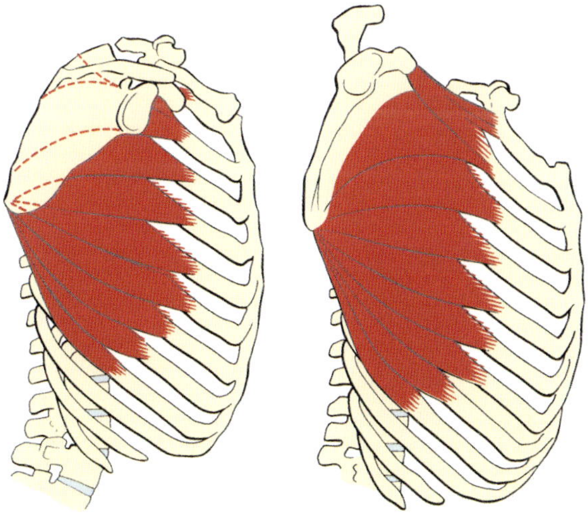

Fig. 68 Serratus anterior. Left: shoulder blade in normal position; right: shoulder blade tilted outwards.

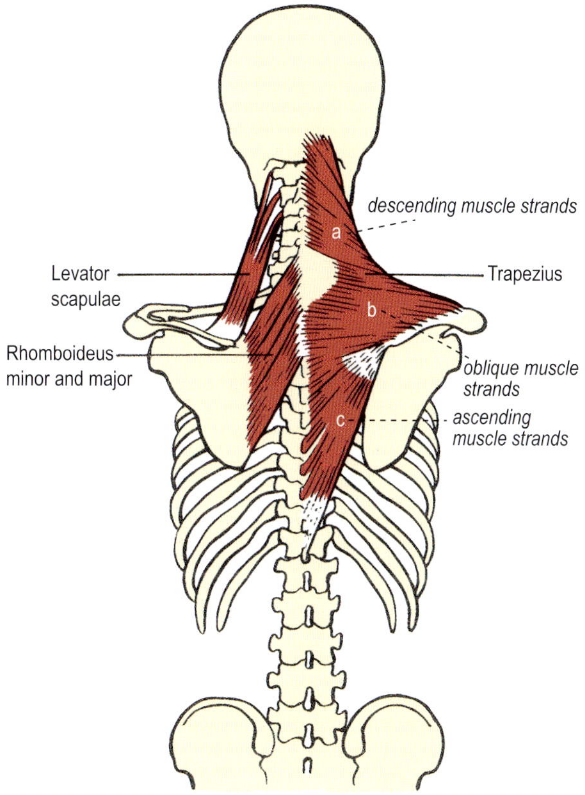

Fig. 69 The dorsal muscles of the shoulder girdle.

This observation is confirmed if one looks at the powerful muscle slings which work together as **agonists** and **antagonists.** It is of fundamental importance that the majority of these muscles firmly integrates the shoulder blade and thus crucially influences its position (and, as a consequence, the position of the whole of the shoulder girdle) (fig. 70).

The following muscle slings are involved:

- the rhomboideus-serratus sling,
- the levator-trapezius sling,
- the trapezius-pectoralis sling and
- the trapezius-serratus sling.

When one looks at the **rhomboideus-serratus sling,** one has the impression that it is a long muscle sling which twists around the thorax with a narrow bony crest formed by the inner margin of the shoulder blade, and which runs obliquely to the traction course of the whole sling:

- if the rhomboids contract, the serrratus anterior is extended at the same time, then the shoulder blade is pulled towards the spine.
- if both of these muscles interchange their function, then the shoulder blade is moved away from the spine.
- if both sections of the sling contract simultaneously, the shoulder blade is fixated in an intermediate position which makes exercises possible and in which the arms support the whole body.

The functional cooperation between the levator scapulae and the ascending muscle strands of the trapezius **(levator-trapezius sling)**, as well as of the transversal parts of the trapezius with the pectoralis minor **(trapezius-pectoralis sling and the trapezius-serratus sling)**, prevents the shoulders from being pushed downwards when carrying heavy loads on the shoulders. The muscle slings shown, which are illustrated in a strictly schematized form in fig. 70, give the shoulder blade and thus the shoulder girdle great mobility in various directions. Without this the arm could not carry out its wide range of movements at the shoulder joint. Moreover, they form the functional-anatomical basis for predominantly **static sequences of movements,** which will be discussed with the help of typical examples from artistic gymnastics, which have achieved a high degree of specialisation as technical and artistic sport disciplines ("apparatus specialists").

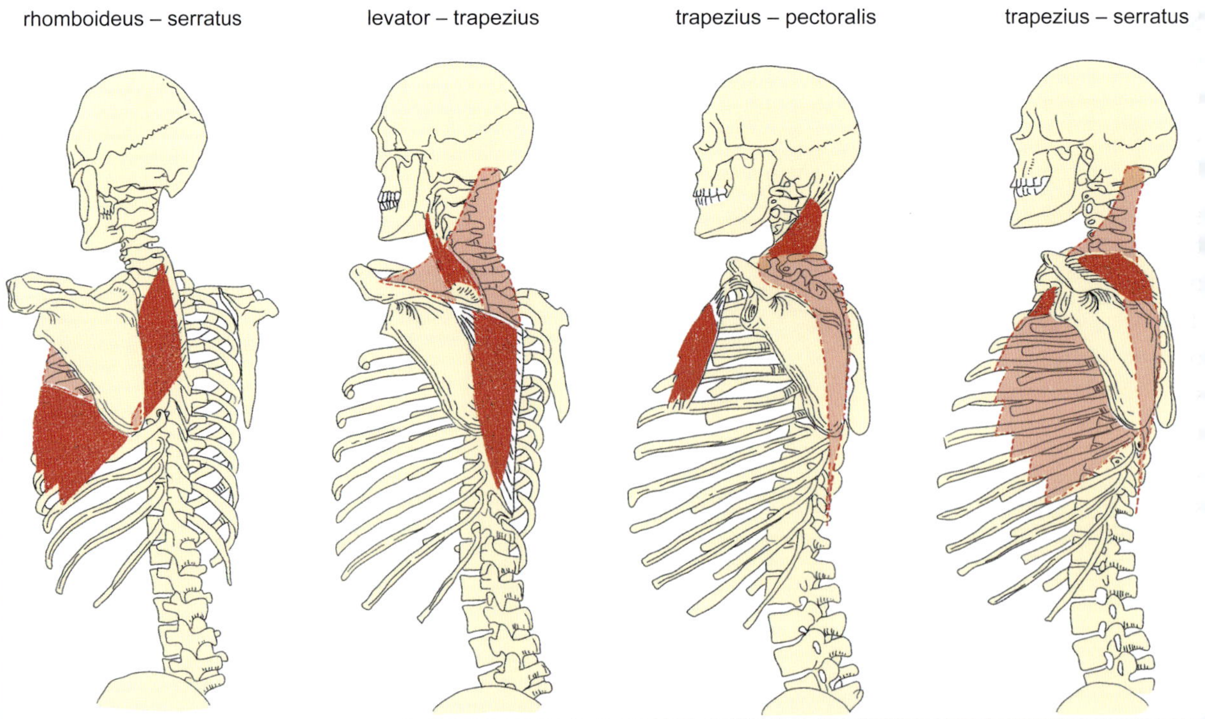

Fig. 70 Schematized illustration of some pairs of muscle which are important for moving and fixating the shoulder blade.

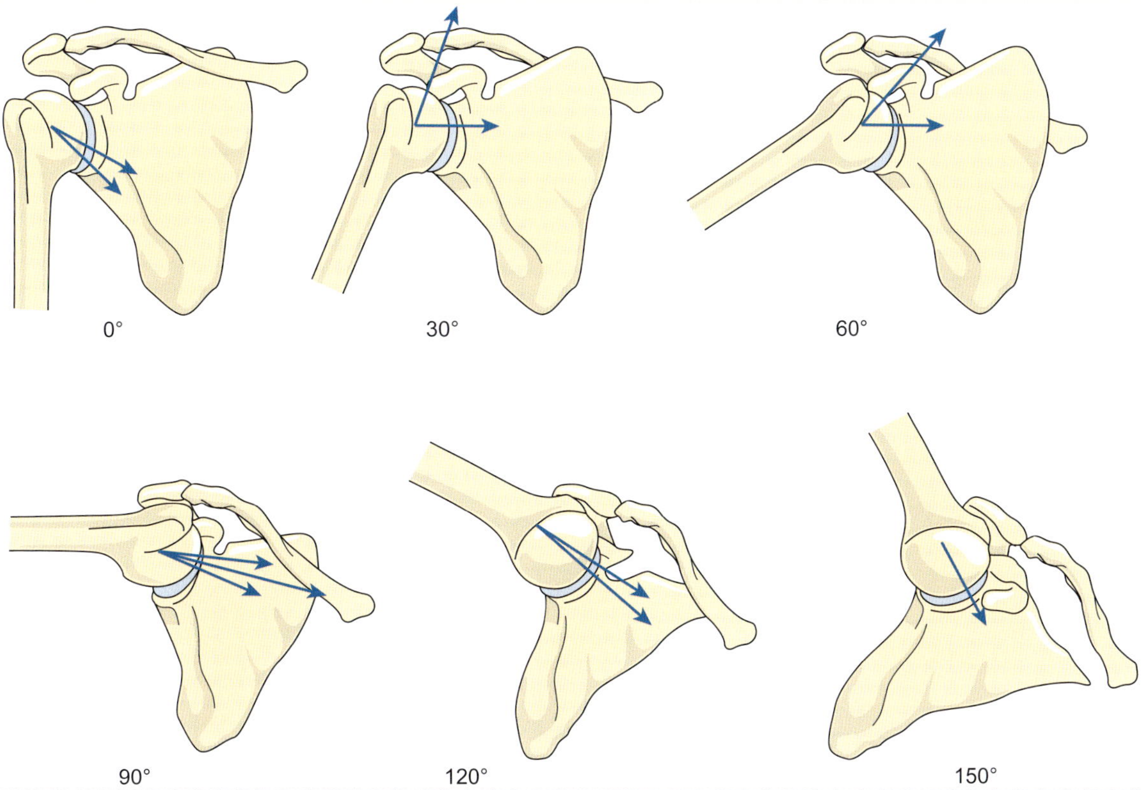

Fig. 71 Schematized illustration of the functional cooperation of shoulder girdle and shoulder joint in various degrees of arm abduction. 0°: starting position, 90°: arm abduction up to 90°, abduction up to 120° or 150°

Static power is the tension which a muscle can exert voluntarily against a fixated object and which is determined by the area of cross-section of all the muscles fibres and by the large number of "fast" muscle fibres (fast-twitch fibres). In exercises in apparatus gymnastics (for example the cross on the rings, the front lever) both static and dynamic demands made on the strength of the athlete.

These examples show that the position and function of the shoulder blade determine the three-dimensional extent of movement at the shoulder joint and upper arm, especially illustrated by the interplay of the serratus-rhomboideus and trapezius-serratus sling (fig. 71 and 72).

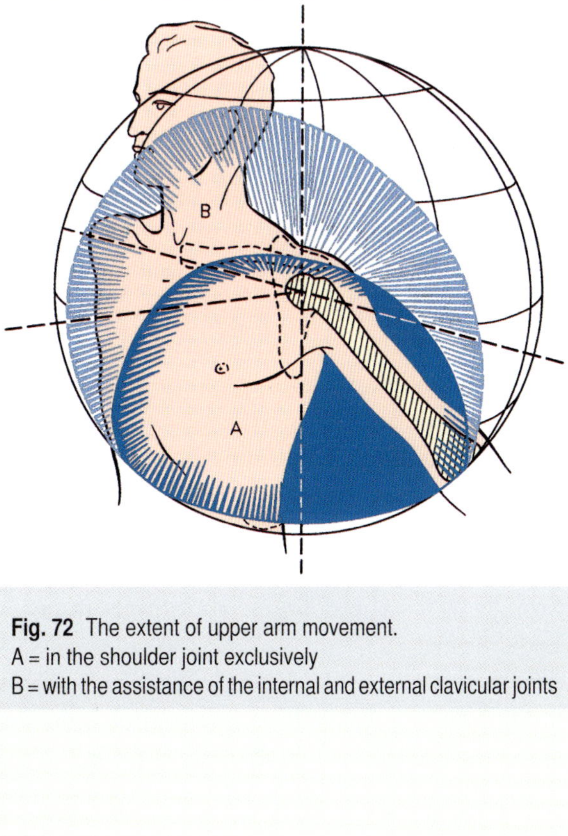

Fig. 72 The extent of upper arm movement.
A = in the shoulder joint exclusively
B = with the assistance of the internal and external clavicular joints

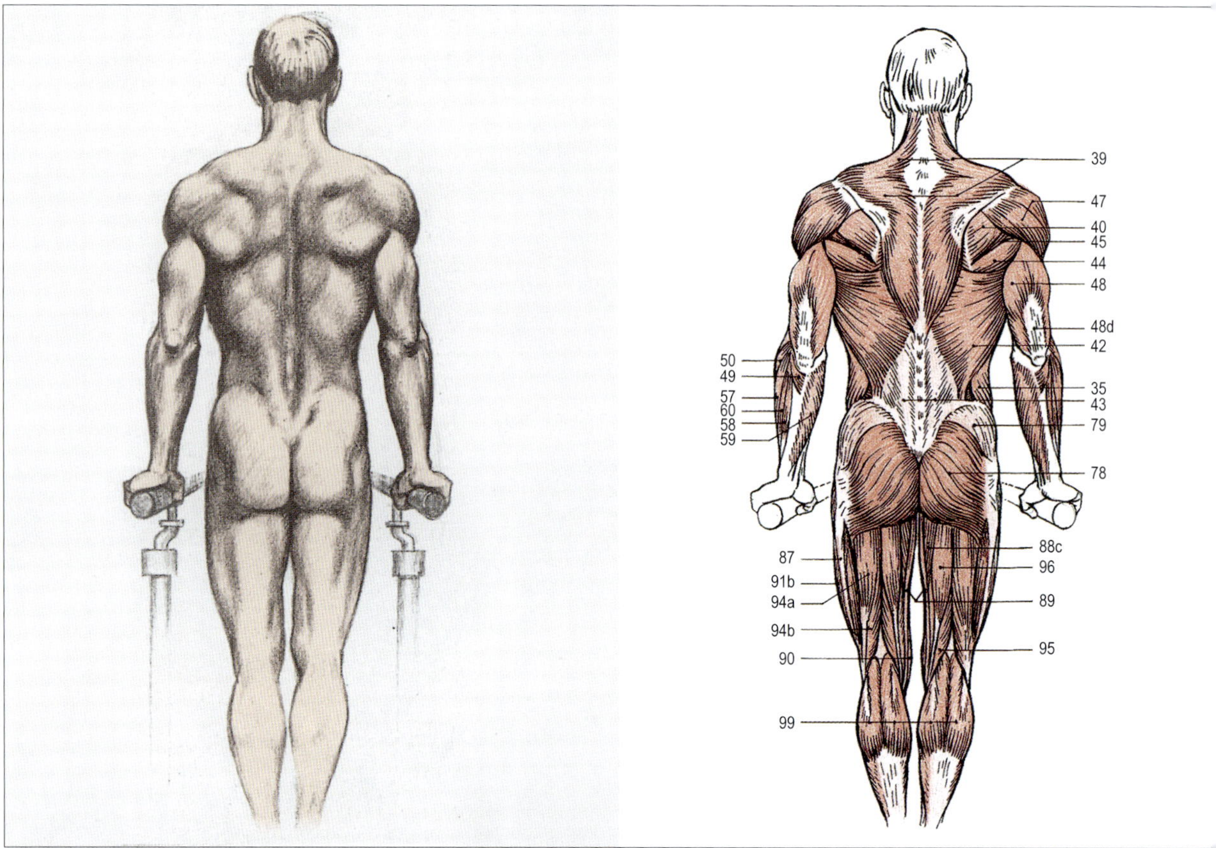

Fig. 73 Muscle slings in the support position on the hands on the parallel bars.

2.5 Muscle slings in static sequences of movements

Gymnast on parallel bars

The illustration (fig. 73) shows a gymnast in the **support position** on the parallel bars. The shoulders are pushed backwards firmly and the inner margins of the shoulder blades which are facing the spine are brought very close to the row of spinal processes. The superficial dorsal muscles, the trapezius and the latissimus dorsi, are clearly visible below the skin, and the aponeurosis of the trapezius as well as the rhomboid fascia thoracolumbalis sink, so to speak, deep below the strongly contracted muscles. In the muscle illustration the lumbar triangle (trigonum lumbale) should be mentioned, through which the obliquus abdominis internus can "shimmer".

The illustrations of the support position – either in the form of a relatively simple support position on the parallel bars or of a **floating support** on the parallel bars (fig. 73, 74a) or the much more difficult **support position on the rings** (fig. 74b) – show that there is a risk of the body sagging between the arms. This can be seen frequently in children in the first school years, whose shoulder girdle muscles are not sufficiently developed. Because the arms, which are extended at the elbow joints, press the head of the humerus and with it the acromion upwards, the shoulder blades swing between the spine, which has a downwards tendency, and the upper extremities, which are pressing upwards.

Which muscles join to form a strong sling which fixates the shoulder girdle in the support position?

These are the **two rhomboid muscles** (major and minor) – supported by the descending and horizontal fibres of the **trapezius** – and the **serratus anterior.**

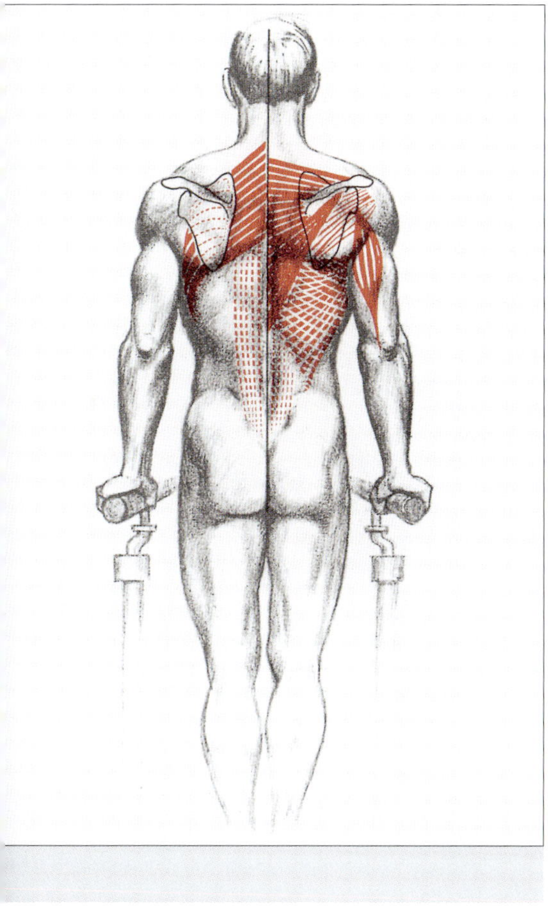

Muscles Fig. 73

- **35** Obliquus externus abdominis
- **39** Trapezius
- **40** Supra- et infraspinatus
- **42** Latissimus dorsi
- **43** Fascia thoracolumbalis
- **44** Teres major
- **45** Teres minor
- **47** Deltoideus
- **48** Triceps brachii
- **48d** Tendon of triceps brachii
- **49** Anconeus
- **50** Biceps brachii
- **57** Extensor carpi radialis brevis
- **58** Extensor carpi ulnaris
- **59** Flexor carpi ulnaris
- **60** Extensor digitorum
- **78** Gluteus maximus
- **79** Gluteus medius
- **87** Tractus iliotibialis
- **88c** Adductor magnus
- **89** Gracilis
- **90** Sartorius
- **91b** Vastus lateralis
- **94a** Biceps femoris, caput longum
- **94b** Biceps femoris, caput breve
- **95** Semimembranosus
- **96** Semitendinosus
- **99** Gastrocnemius

- If the fibres are shortened in one part of the rhomboideus-serratus sling, then there is, at the same time, an equally pronounced extension of the other part.
- If both parts contract at the same time, then there is a powerful fixation of the shoulder blade, and thus of the whole shoulder girdle.

n this position the **rhomboideus-serratus sling ecomes the weight-bearer of the whole body.** f this sling slackens, then the body loses its firm, ecure posture, the arms press the acromion upwards nd the trunk sags under its own weight.

There is a specific problem with the sequence of novements illustrated, which affects the techni-al-artistic sport disciplines and the mutual influ-nce of high-power demands and extreme-mobility mplitude. The rapid-power elements which have

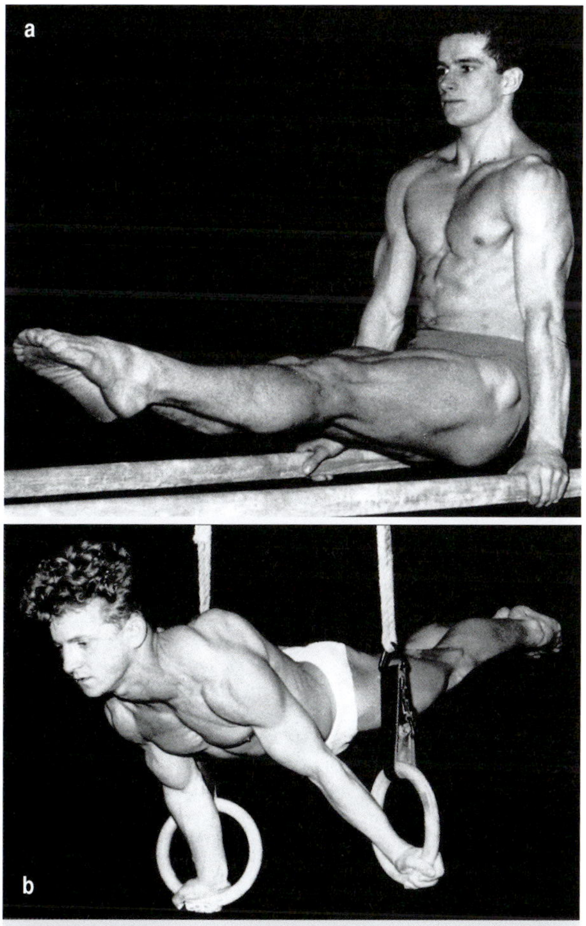

Fig. 74 Holding the legs in a horizontal position on the parallel bars (a) and on the rings (b).

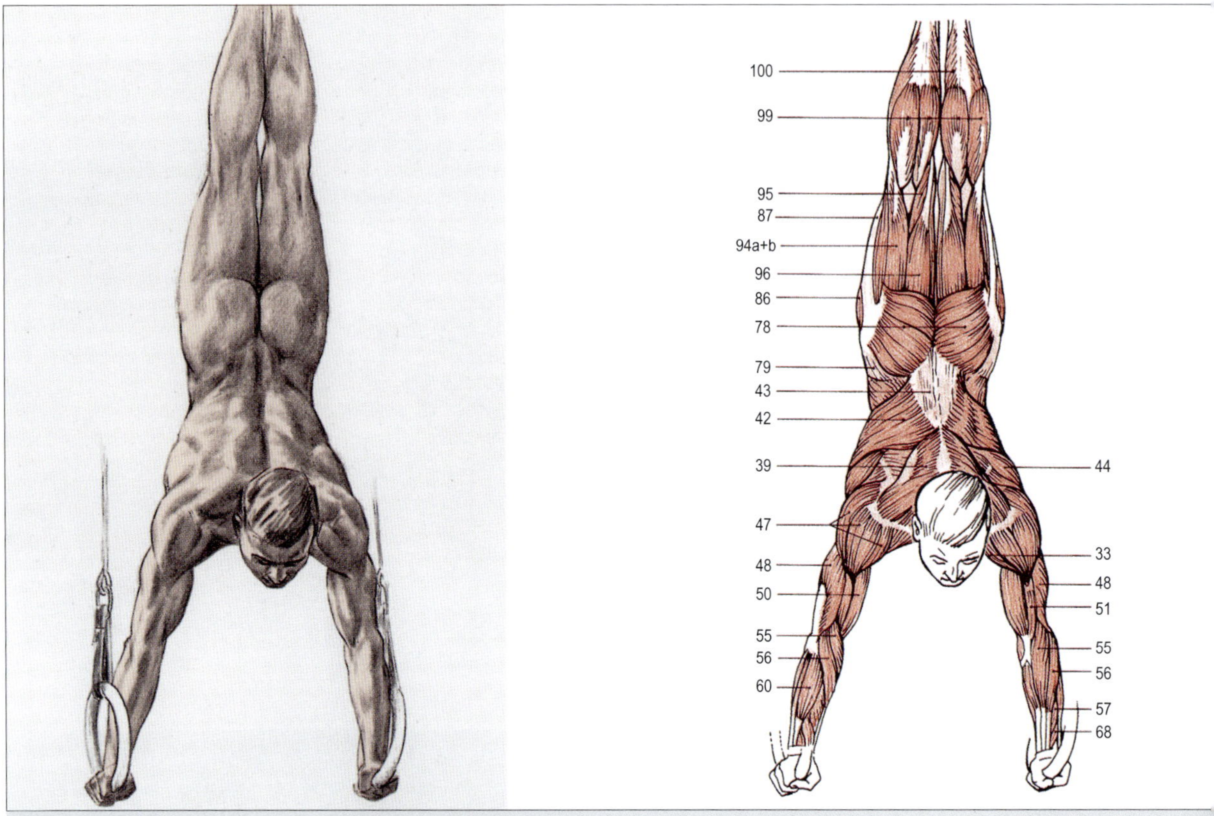

Fig. 75 Muscles slings in a gymnast doing a handstand on the steady rings.

been trained lead to a significant **shortening of the powerful muscles** in the muscle sling, and, at the same time, to a reduction of their elasticity, which inevitably leads to a **muscular imbalance,** and thus to a disturbance of the coordination of movements and to an insufficient and imprecise mobility. This is often the cause of injury to a muscle or tendon. It is worth noticing in this context that the sling described flows into the **obliquus abdominis externus** on the same side, which will be discussed in greater detail in one of the next sequences of movements. The deep dorsal muscles as well as the extensors of the upper and lower extremities become part of the whole-body sling as more or less supporting links.

Gymnast on the rings

After having demonstrated the front-lever position with the legs in a horizontal position, it is very interesting to have a look at a **handstand on the steady rings** (fig. 75), which has now been modified by developing the power and swinging elements into a cross support, and on the parallel bars (fig. 76). In an exercise of this kind which, in order to maintain body equilibrium, puts a great strain on the strength and strength endurance of the arms, the shoulder girdle, the trunk and the lumbar spine, the shoulder blade (and with it the shoulder girdle as a whole) are pressed towards the pelvis. While the shoulder blade in the support position extends with its lower angle into the recess of the latissimus dorsi, in the handstand on the rings and on the parallel bar

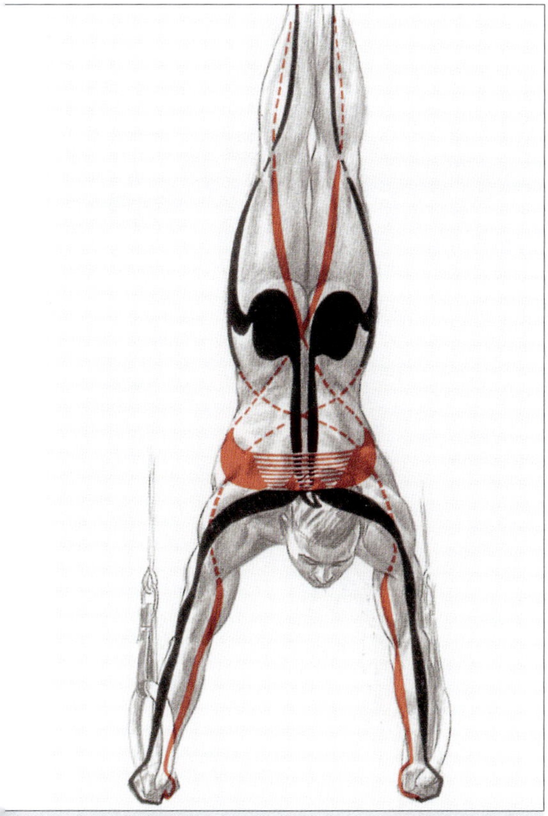

Muscles Fig. 75

33 Pectoralis major
39 Trapezius
42 Latissimus dorsi
43 Fascia thoracolumbalis
44 Teres major
47 Deltoideus
48 Triceps brachii
50 Biceps brachii
51 Brachialis
55 Brachioradialis
56 Extensor carpi radialis longus
57 Extensor carpi radialis brevis
60 Extensor digitorum
68 Abductor pollicis longus
78 Gluteus maximus
79 Gluteus medius
86 Tensor fasciae latae
87 Tractus iliotibialis
94a Biceps femoris, caput longum
94b Biceps femoris, caput breve
95 Semimembranosus
96 Semitendinosus
99 Gastrocnemius
100 Soleus

ts lower edge protrudes. The rhomboids and the serratus anterior, which run in the same direction when the body is in a stationary position (see fig. 70 and 73), now extend towards the shoulder blade in an acute angle. Securing the handstand depends on their mutual coordination because they determine the position of the cavity of the shoulder joint on the head of the humerus with their powerful muscle contraction. **The rhomboideus-serratus sling holds the body,** even in a handstand, **like a broad, powerful muscular girdle,** which extends from the spine via the ribs and the obliquus externus muscles (their stabilizing effect should be particularly emphasized) to the pelvis.

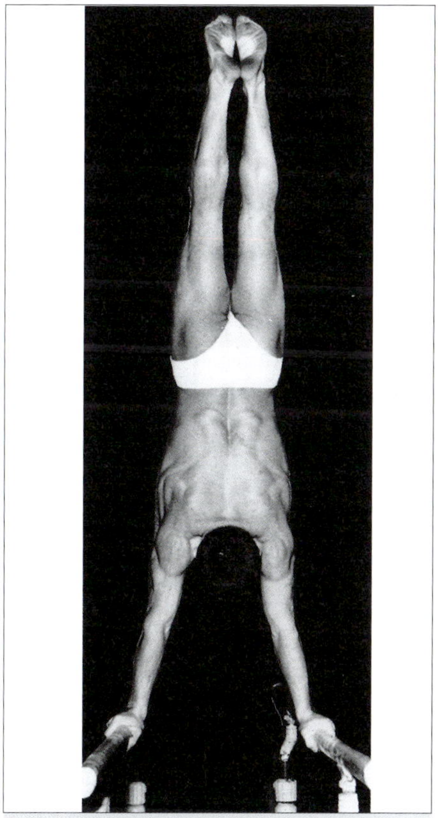

Fig. 76 Handstand on the parallel bars.

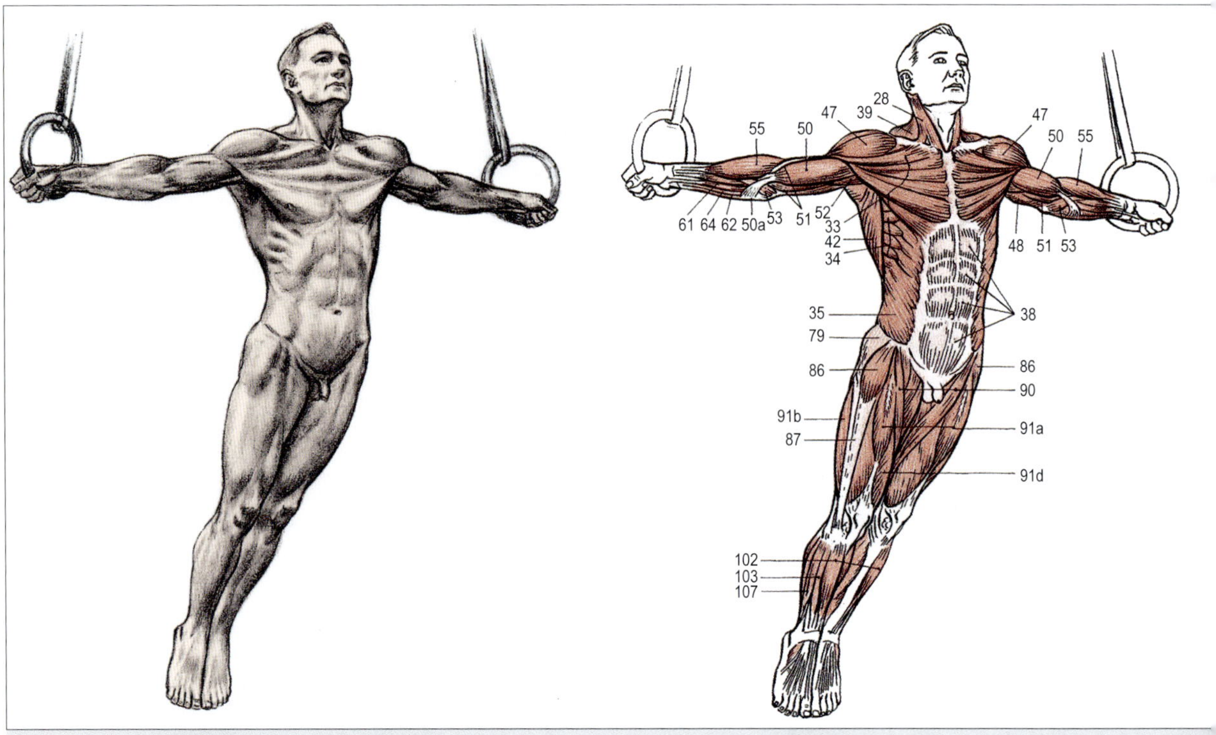

Fig. 77 Muscle slings in a gymnast in the cross support.

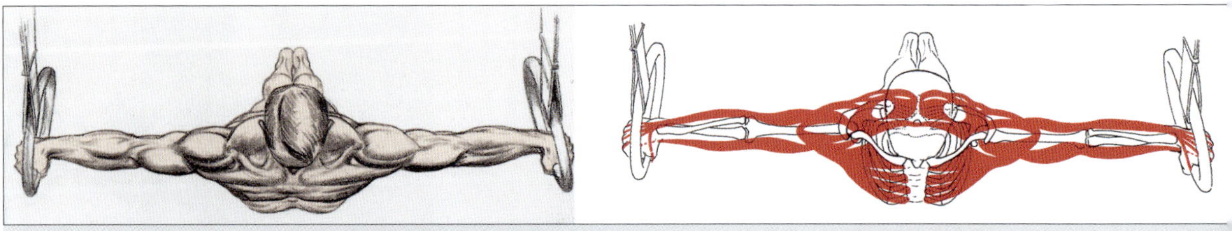

Fig. 78 Muscle slings in a gymnast in the cross support (seen from above).

The next illustrations, the cross support on the rings (fig. 77–79) show clearly what enormous demands are made on the gymnast's strength in carrying out this sequence of movements which have always been a highlight of apparatus gymnastics. To achieve this the following training methods are required:

- **maximum-power** training with predominantly static-power exertion (with virtually no movement), which forms the basis for static-power elements on the floor, on the parallel bars and on the rings,
- the training of **fast power,** which is importan for the coordination of power impulses of varying degrees, for upswings, jumps with multipl whole-body rotations along the vertical or horizontal axis and for take-off and push-off movements of the upper extremities and
- **power-endurance** training (in exercises lastin up to 1.5 min).

This variety underlines the importance of th **complexity of power training** as well as the uni

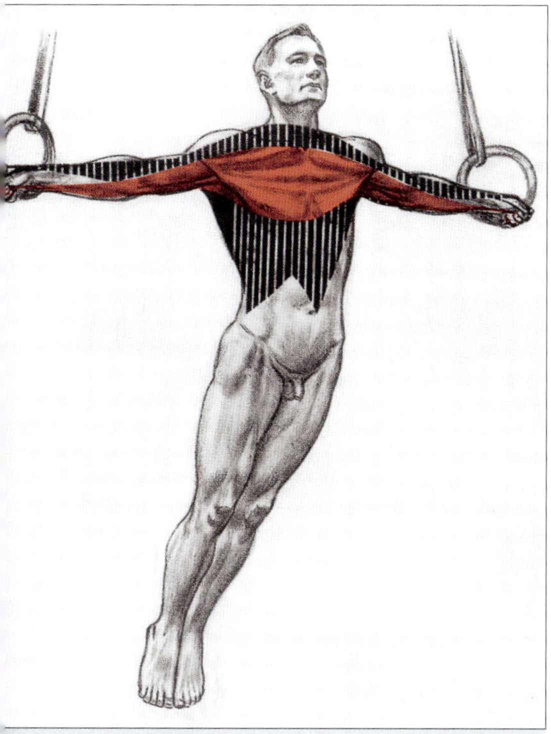

Muscles Fig. 77
28 Sternocleidomastoideus
33 Pectoralis major
34 Serratus anterior
35 Obliquus externus abdominis
38 Rectus abdominis
39 Trapezius
42 Latissimus dorsi
47 Deltoideus
48 Triceps brachii
50 Biceps brachii
50a Aponeurosis bicipitis brachii
51 Brachialis
52 Coracobrachialis
53 Pronator teres
55 Brachioradialis
61 Flexor carpi radialis
62 Flexor digitorum superficialis
64 Palmaris longus
79 Gluteus medius
86 Tensor fasciae latae
87 Tractus iliotibialis
90 Sartorius
91a Rectus femoris
91b Vastus lateralis
91d Vastus intermedius
102 Tibialis anterior
103 Extensor digitorum longus
107 Fibularis longus

ied development of capabilities and skills (pow-
er and technique). The stepwise **development of maximal-power potentials** in the shoulder and pelvic girdles is a crucial precondition for the application of differentiated muscular power which is necessary, for example, for the support scales, the hang scales, and the cross support, following on from complicated sequences of movements on different kinds of apparatus. The work potential of the responsible adductors and abductors of the upper arm at the shoulder joint as well as the

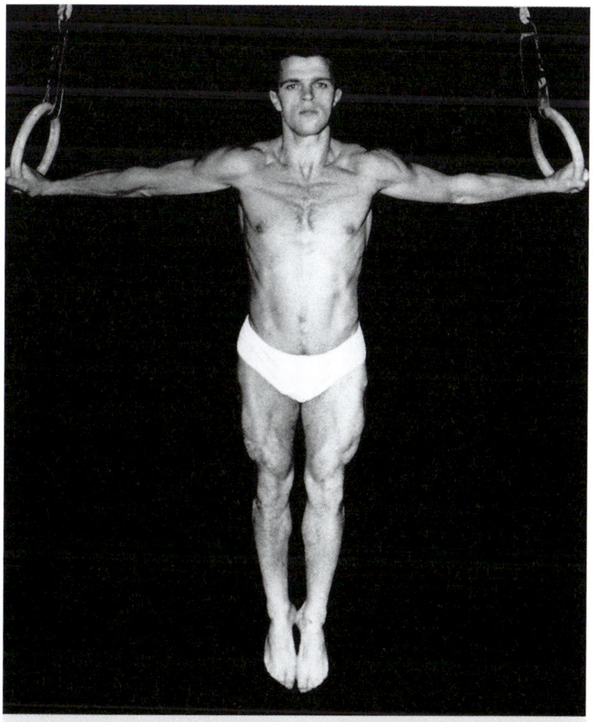

Fig. 79 Cross support on the rings.

flexors of the thigh at the hip joint are shown in tables 13–15.

Table 13: Work potential of the adductors of the upper arm at the shoulder joint of 96°, from 88° abduction to 8° adduction.

	kg/m
Deltoid muscle, anterior section	3.0
Deltoid muscle, posterior section	0.4
Subscapularis	1.0
Pectoralis major, sternum-rib section	9.9
Pectoralis major, clavicular section	1.4
Pectoralis major, abdominal fascia section	0.5
Infraspinatus	0.2
Teres minor	0.1
Coracobrachialis	2.0
Teres major	7.3
Biceps brachii, long head	2.1
Latissimus dorsi, superior part	3.3
Latissimus dorsi, inferior part	2.2
Triceps brachii, long head	8.5
All Adductors	41.9

Table 14: Work potential of the abductors of the upper arm at the shoulder joint of 96°, from 8° adduction, to 88° abduction.

	kg/m
Deltoid muscle, middle section	12.1
Deltoid muscle, anterior section	0.3
Deltoid muscle, posterior section	0.5
Supraspinatus	3.6
Infraspinatus	2.9
Subscapularis	0.2
Teres minor	0.1
Biceps brachii, long head	1.2
All Abductors	20.9

Table 15: Work potential of the flexors of the thigh at the hip joint.

	kg/m
Rectus femoris	19.4
Tensor fasciae latae	7.5
Sartorius	4.8
Iliopsoas	14.3
Pectineus	2.9
Adductor femoris longus	1.6
Adductor femoris magnus	1.3
Gracilis	0.1
Gluteus minimus	3.5
All flexors (including obturatorius externus, Adductor femoris brevis and quadratus femoris)	> 55.4

It is obvious, after these introductory remarks, which muscles groups do the main work in this difficult exercise, which requires great power. As in the support position on the parallel bars or in the handstand on the steady rings, it is important, above all, **to fixate the shoulder girdle and shoulder joint** – which is much more complicated in the cross support compared to the movements we are already familiar with. Like the strong iron rings which hold a wine barrel together, to prevent the pieces of damp wood from swelling and coming apart, the following muscles hold the **back of the trunk** in the cross support:

- the rhomboids
- the serratus anterior
- the obliquus abdominis externus
- the trapezius
- the latissimus dorsi and
- the deltoid,

and the pectoralis major with its sternal, rib and clavicular sections and the **front of the trunk,** as fig. 79 and 80 demonstrate.

In this context the **functional cooperation between pectoralis major and latissimus dorsi,** which are both muscles of the shoulder joint, should be emphasized. The large "physiological cross-section" of both extensive muscles, which represents the sum of the areas of all the muscles fibres which have been cut vertically to their length (see below), makes it possible not only to move the arm at the shoulder joint (as agonists and antagonists) forwards and backwards (ante- and retroversion), but also for these extensive muscles to move the trunk towards the arm. For this reason they play an important part in **holding the arm close to the trunk.** Both muscles adduct the arm and thus hold the shoulder girdle firmly to the trunk, when the trunk is about to sag under heavy loads. Moreover both muscles are powerful internal and external rotators. The adductors and internal rotators of the arm are on the whole stronger than their antagonists. This makes it possible for them **not only to fixate the shoulder girdle, but also to work against a load or against the body,** whereas the antagonists only have to move the weight of the arm.

! A few remarks on the "physiological cross section" of a skeletal muscle: if the muscle fibres run lengthwise, then the size of the physiological cross-section depends on the number of actin and myosin filaments in the muscle. If the area of the cross-section is 6 cm^2, then the maximum contractile power is 6 x 49 N = 294 N. If the muscle fibres run obliquely to the longitudinal direction of the whole muscle (as in a singly or doubly feathered muscle), then the total physiological cross-section (especially in the case of the doubly feathered muscle), because of the addition of two cross sectional areas (6 cm^2 each), is 12 cm^2 and there is a maximum power (12 x 49 N) of 588 N. Feathered muscles are as a consequence significantly more powerful, although their muscle mass can be the same as that of a fusiform muscle.

In addition to the upper-arm adductors at the shoulder joint, whose work potential (in kg/m) can be looked up in table 13, the following muscles are also involved in the sequence of movements described above:

- the long head of the triceps brachii,
- the teres major,
- the coracobrachialis as well as
- the subscapularis.

One has the impression that **the body is hanging in a very strong muscle ring** (fig. 78) and that the correct performance of the cross support on the rings depends on its contractile power. All the other muscles in the region of the upper and lower extremities have a merely more or less supportive function. The comparison which was made with a wine barrel or with its iron rings, seems therefore to be justified, as the latter closely resemble in their form and function the muscle girdle of the trunk. This can be seen by looking down, from a higher point of view, on the gymnast performing the cross support, as shown in fig. 79.

Another very exhausting, difficult exercise is the cross support on the rings with the legs extended horizontally forwards (fig. 80). In addition to the above-mentioned muscle groups or muscle slings for the fixation of the shoulder girdle and the shoulder joint, in this case the **flexors of the thigh at the hip joint (tab. 15) and parts of the abdominal muscles are maximally contracted.** One can see, for example, the powerfully contracted quadriceps femoris as well as the bulging tensor fasciae latae on the body surface.

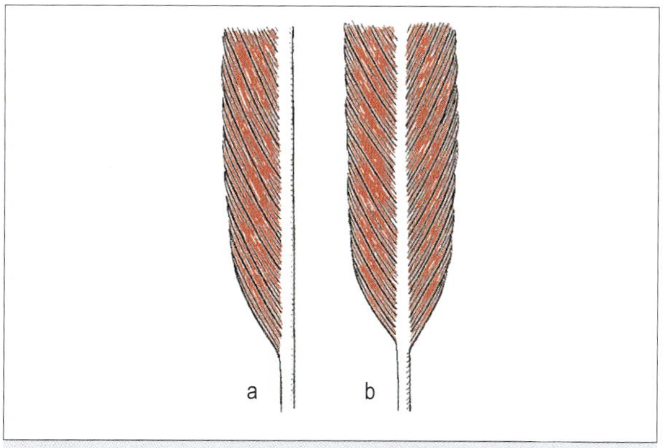

Fig. 79a Singly and doubly feathered muscles. Examples:
a: fibularis brevis, extensor digitorum longus, extensor hallucis longus,
b: rectus femoris, tibialis anterior, flexor carpi radialis, palmaris longus.

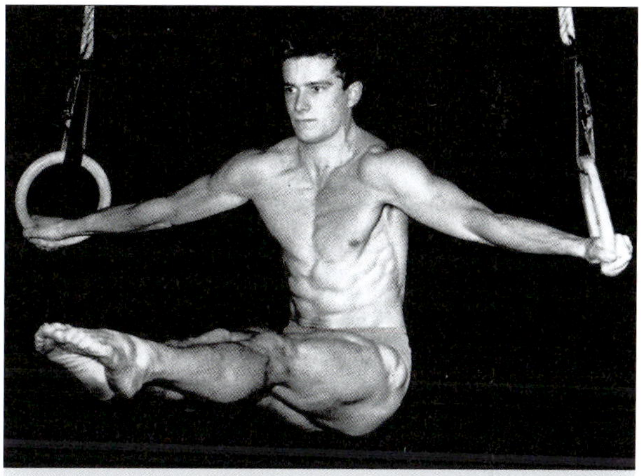

Fig. 80 The cross support on the rings with the legs extended forwards.

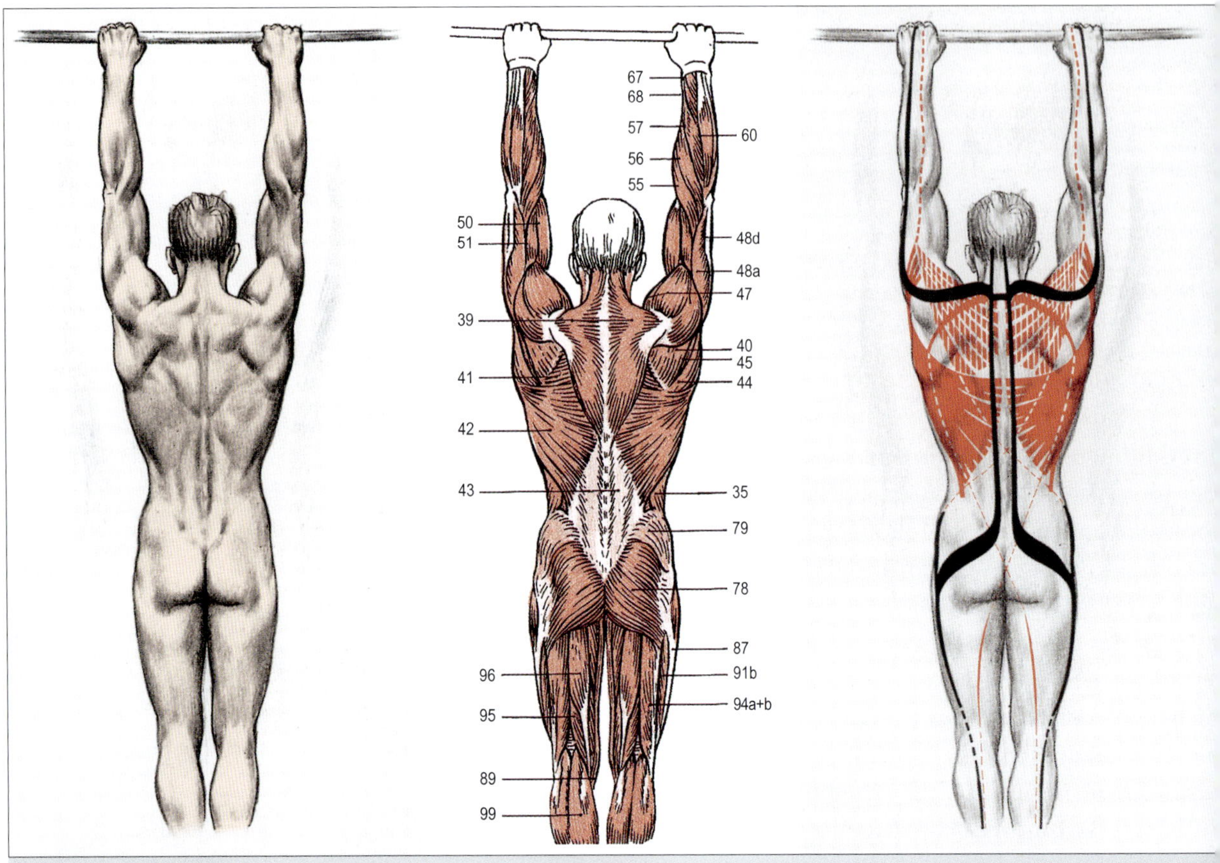

Fig. 81 Muscle slings in a gymnast hanging from the high bar.

High-bar gymnast

The muscle-sling illustration of the hanging position with extended arms from the high bar (fig. 81), which is the initial position for many exercises on the high bar, is intended to show how the body, as in the cross support, is kept in equilibrium by the already-mentioned powerful muscle combination of the **pectoralis major and the latissimus dorsi.** Both muscles enable the athlete to pull his body from a hanging position of maximal extension, on the 240 cm long and 28 mm in diameter high bar, upwards to the pull-up position. This is achieved by the cooperation of the three lower arm flexors at the elbow joint (fig. 82): the **biceps brachii, the brachialis and the brachioradialis.** This flexion is carried out most effectively if the lower arm is supinated (not seen in the illustration).

The particularly well developed ability, compared with other muscles, to extend the pectoralis major and the latissimus dorsi is due to the fact that the muscle strands originating from the lowest level on the trunk insert at the highest level on the upper arm. The **fibres of the final section of the muscle** which are inserted into the bone, **are wrapped-up.** This has the advantage that even when the arm is

Muscles Fig. 81
- **35** Obliquus externus abdominis
- **39** Trapezius
- **40** Supra- et infraspinatus
- **41** Rhomboideus major
- **42** Latissimus dorsi
- **43** Fascia thoracolumbalis
- **44** Teres major
- **45** Teres minor
- **47** Deltoideus
- **48a** Caput laterale m. tricipitis brachii
- **48d** Tendon of triceps brachii
- **50** Biceps brachii
- **51** Brachialis
- **55** Brachioradialis
- **56** Extensor carpi radialis longus
- **57** Extensor carpi radialis brevis
- **60** Extensor digitorum
- **67** Extensor pollicis brevis
- **68** Abductor pollicis longus
- **78** Gluteus maximus
- **79** Gluteus medius
- **87** Tractus iliotibialis
- **89** Gracilis
- **91b** Vastus lateralis
- **94a+b** Caput longum, caput breve, biceps femoris
- **95** Semimembranosus
- **96** Semitendinosus
- **99** Gastrocnemius

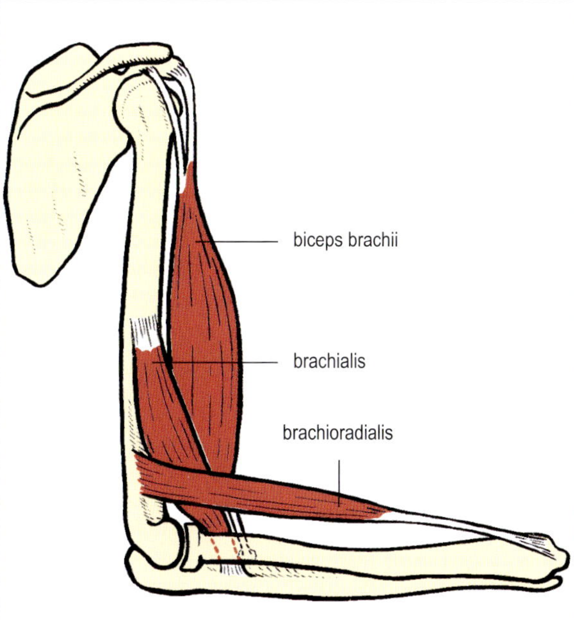

Fig. 82 The flexors of the lower arm at the elbow joint.

hanging down they can exert an influence on the arm and bring the hand towards the abdomen or the pelvis. When the arm is raised and the muscles are unwrapped (fig. 83), then the muscles fibres run in parallel in the same direction. Their relatively long course, when the arm is hanging downwards, now becomes shorter.

! These examples once again make it clear that the output of a muscle cannot be evaluated solely from the interdependent relationship between its points of origin and insertion. No movement of our body is an isolated phenomenon because it must always be understood and assessed in the context of its functional relationship to the whole.

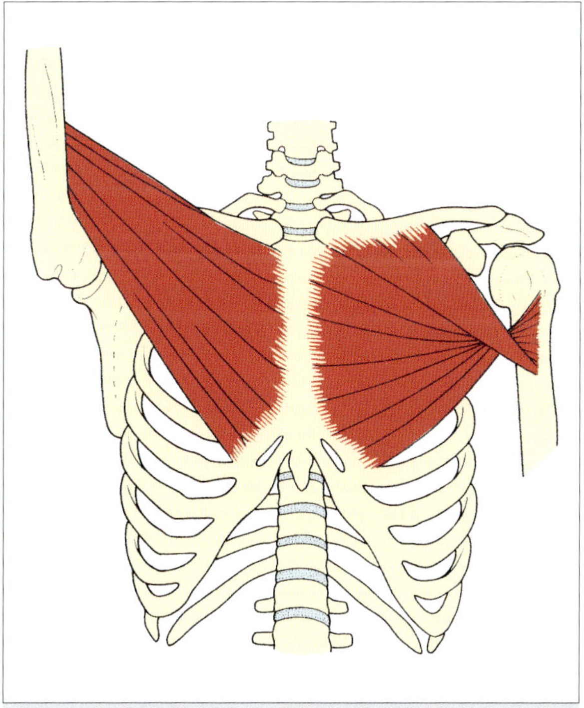

Fig. 83 Pectoralis major: Crossing-over of the fibre strands before the point of insertion at rest and the unwinding of the fibres when the arm is raised.

Role and integration of the abdominal muscles in lateral inclination and rotation

The role of the abdominal muscles within longer muscle slings extending over the whole body has already been emphasized in the analyses of dynamic and static sequences of movements in sport. This applies particularly to all the movements of the spine. When we now turn to the lateral inclination and rotation of the trunk, these cannot be understood without adequate knowledge of the structure of the abdominal muscles, of the cooperation of their individual components and of their integration in the different muscle slings. For this reason the structure of the abdominal wall, which is of great importance in the following sequences of movements, will now be briefly described.

The large space between the lower opening of the thoracic cage, the upper edge of the pelvis and the lumbar spine is filled by a powerful wide, elastic and adjustable, multi-layered **muscular-tendinous girdle,** which extends from the lumbar spine to the midline of the body. Because of its connection with the ribs this girdle is able to transfer movements, for example anterior or lateral inclination or rotation, to the central axial skeleton.

This **muscular and aponeurotic system,** which has in its anterior and lateral region a crosswise "rigging" of its individual components (fig. 84), resulting in an increased resistance, **is composed of the following muscles:**

- the obliquus abdominis externus
- the obliquus abdominis internus
- the transversus abdominis
- the rectus abdominis
- the pyramidalis and
- the quadratus lumborum.

The obliquus abdominis externus (fig. 84) originates from a broad base with 8 fleshy spikes from the outer surface of the 5th to the 12th rib, and extends obliquely from cranial posterior to caudal anterior into a broad tendinous plate (aponeurosis) the fibrous components of which cross in the midline of the body with those from the other side. Its **function** is, in the case of unilateral contraction of the muscle fibres, the powerful inclining of the trunk towards the same side. If the right and left external oblique muscles contract simultaneously, then there is a forward inclination of the trunk (when the pelvis is fixated at the same time).

The obliquus abdominis internus (fig. 84), which lies below the outer oblique abdominal muscle, originates from the superficial layer of the fascia

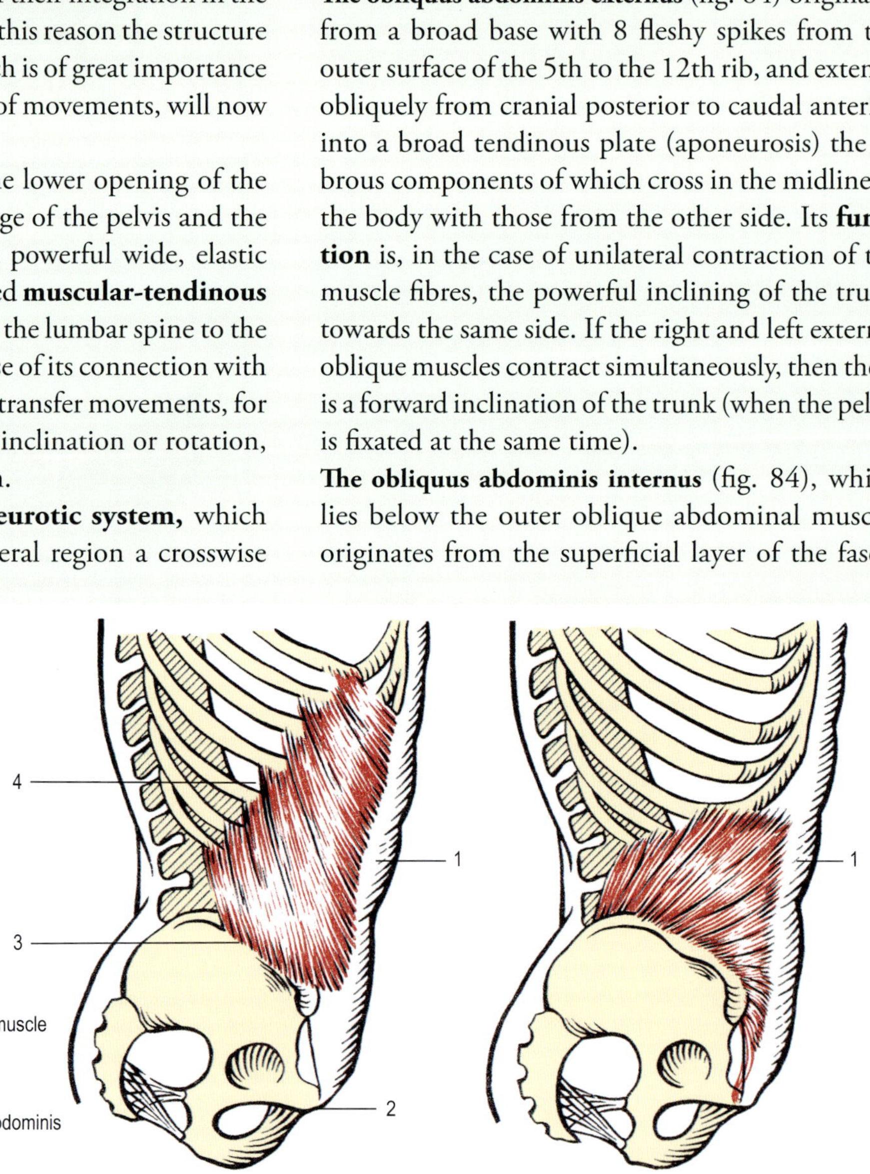

1 Aponeurosis of the obliquus abdominis externus and internus muscle
2 Pubic bone (Os pubis)
3 Outer rim of the iliac crest (Labium externum cristae iliacae)
4 Originating area of the obliquus abdominis externus from the lower 8 ribs

Fig. 84 The outer (left) and inner (right) oblique abdominal muscle (M. obliquus abdominis externus and internus).

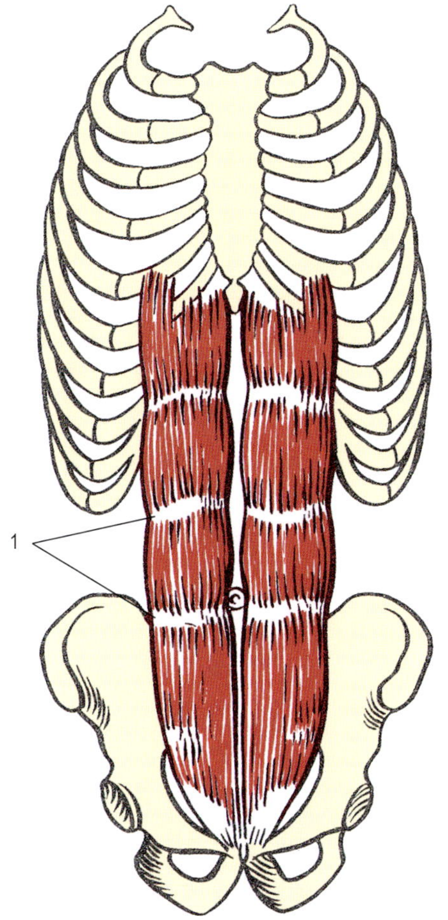

1 Tendinous intersections in the muscle (intersectiones tendineae)

Fig. 85 The Rectus abdominis.

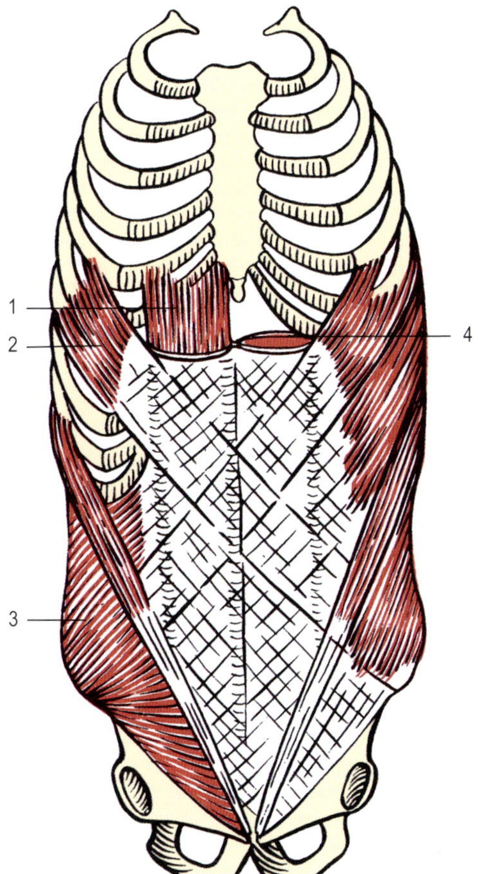

1 Rectus abdominis
2 Obliquus abdominis externus
3 Obliquus abdominis internus now visible because the obliquus externus in this area has been largely removed on the right side of the body.
4 Rectus sheath (Vagina m. recti abdominis)

Fig. 86 Schematic picture of the muscles which build up abdominal muscle pressure.

thoracolumbalis, from the crest of the iliac bones as well as from the inguinal ligament, and extends in its further course, like a fan:

- the posterior muscle strands run upwards to the last three ribs
- the middle components run obliquely and horizontally to the midline of the body and
- the anterior strands run from the cremaster muscle and downwards to the spermatic cord.

The middle strands of the inner oblique abdominal muscle, which do not insert at the ribs, cross under the strands of the outer oblique abdominal muscle at an approximately right angle, and their final sections join the aponeurosis. The latter divides into an anterior and posterior layer at the **edge of the rectus abdominis** (fig. 85–87), forms a sheath around it and thus constitutes the major part of the so-called **rectus sheath** (fig. 86). **Function:** When

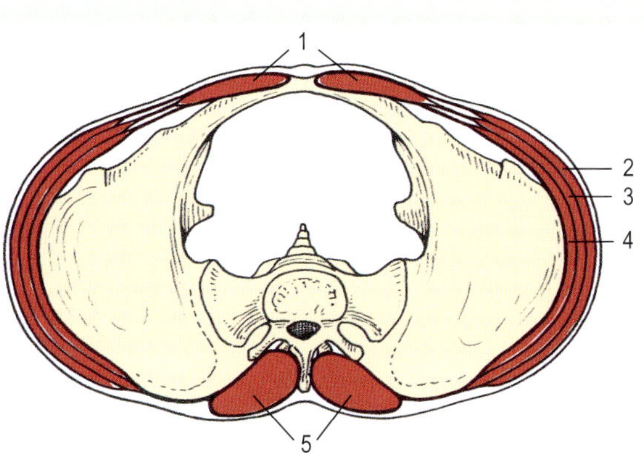

1 Rectus abdominis
2 Obliquus abdominis externus
3 Obliquus abdominis internus
4 Transversus abdominis
5 Erector spinae

Fig. 87 Cross-section of the wall of the trunk (at the level of the navel).

contracted **unilaterally,** the trunk is inclined to the same side and rotated by the inner oblique muscle. This happens in cooperation with the outer oblique abdominal muscle of the other side, which is drawn towards it. This will be described in detail later. If the inner oblique muscles contract **bilaterally**, then they draw the ribs forwards and downwards and thus **flex the trunk forwards,** when the pelvis is fixated.

The transversus abdominis (fig. 88), which lies underneath the external and internal oblique abdominal muscles, originates from the inner surfaces of the 7th to the 12th rib, from the deep layer of the fascia thoracolumbalis, from the crest of the iliac bone and from the inguinal ligament. Then it runs obliquely forwards and merges into the aponeurosis. With regard to the directions of their fibres, the right and left oblique abdominal muscles can be compared to **a broad abdominal band which makes the waistline visible when contracted powerfully.** The **function** of the muscle, when contracted bilaterally, is to constrict the abdominal cavity and its contents (abdominal muscle pressure) by pulling the ribs, from which it mainly originates, inwards.

The rectus abdominis (fig. 85–87), which runs along both sides of the midline of the body, originates from the outer surface of the 5th to the 7th rib and from the xiphoid process of the sternum, and then runs caudally with its parallel fibres and inserts with a strong tendon into the area of the symphysis. This long muscle has 3–4, up to 1 cm high, tendinous intersections (intersectiones tendineae) which can be observed in a well-trained athlete (fig. 74a, 77 and 80) in the form of deep grooves on the anterior abdominal wall ("six-pack"). Between these the individual components of the rectus abdominis bulge out when contracted powerfully, as can clearly be seen in the illustrations mentioned. This is because the tendinous intersections are tightly connected to the anterior wall of the rectus sheath. Both muscles are prevented laterally from coming apart by the tendinous structure. The function of the muscle is to raise and support the pelvis when the pelvis is not fixated (for example when hanging from wall bars or during an upward circle on the horizontal bar). When the pelvis is fixated (when the points of origin and insertion are interchanged), the trunk is inclined anteriorly, for example when the upper part of the body is raised from a supine position. This movement is supported by the iliopsoas, acting as a synergist. **This makes the rectus abdominis the most important antagonist of the deep short and long muscles of the back. It is also important for the fixation of the trunk when lifting and carrying heavy weights.**

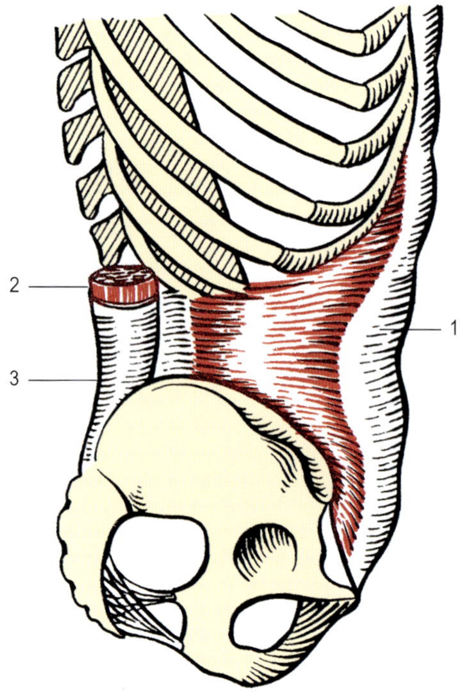

1 Aponeurosis of the oblique abdominal muscle
2 The deep long muscles of the back (erector spinae)
3 Their aponeurosis

Fig. 88 The transversus abdominis.

The pyramidalis and the quadratus lumborum

The narrow pyramidalis muscle originates from the symphysis; it is only weakly developed in humans, spans the midline of the body and is of no great importance for the movement of the trunk. The quadratus lumborum, which constitutes the posterior abdominal muscles, extends from the iliac crest, where it originates, to the 12th rib (and the transversal processes of the lumbar vertebrae) (fig. 52). Its **function** is to draw the 12th rib caudally, which, by **bilateral contraction,** secures the lumbar lordosis and supports the trunk to adjust the body equilibrium. When **unilaterally contracted** the muscle contributes to the ipsilateral inclination of the trunk.

As already mentioned, the two rectus muscles are :ucked like a sword in a sheath which is formed ike a quiver by the aponeuroses of the lateral ab-dominal muscles, for which the aponeurosis of the nner oblique abdominal muscle forms the base with its anterior and posterior layer (fig. 86 and 39). The two other abdominal muscles are involved n stengthening the rectus sheath (Vagina m. recti abdominis): the aponeurosis of the external oblique abdominal muscle merges into the anterior lamella, he aponeurosis of the oblique abdominal muscles nerges into the posterior lamella of the sheath. In his way both of the rectus muscles are fixated in heir position, and, apart from this, linked with the other abdominal muscles to bring about a common effect – which is the **crucial point!** In this context we refer to an oblique, longitudinal and transversal abdominal muscular belt, which can be compared o the plywood principle, according to which the naximum performance and a high degree of pres-sure and traction are achieved with a minimum of naterial (fig. 89).

f one considers, in conclusion, the total perfor-nance of the anterior, lateral and posterior abdom-nal muscles, **they have a crucial influence** on the oosture and movement of the pelvis and the spine, and thus **on the movement of the whole body,** for which the big and long lever arms are advantageous. The longitudinal, oblique and transversal belts of he abdominal muscles (fig. 89) never operate as ndividual anatomical structures, because they are connected to the rectus sheath. They are to be un-lerstood as a very important part of a higher system, especially as the abdominal muscles as a functional unity are part of the large muscle slings, which connect the trunk with the upper and lower extremities. This special structure and function of the abdominal muscles is crucial for the analysis of the following sequences of movements in sport, since the majority of the total body slings make use, above all, of the oblique belt of the abdominal muscles.

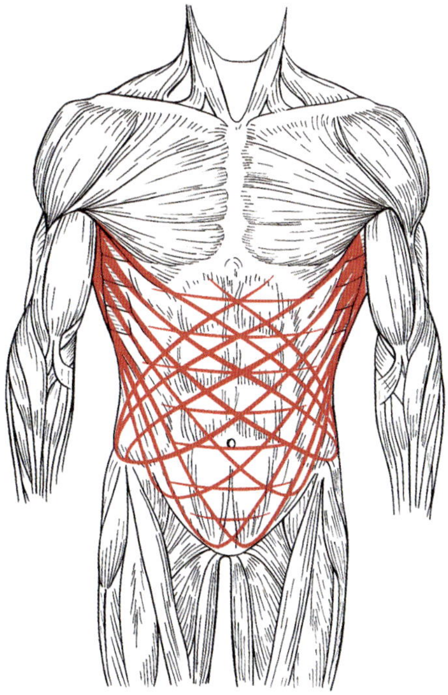

Fig. 89 Schematic illustration of the transverse and oblique belt of the abdominal wall.

2.6 Muscle slings in lateral inclination and rotation of the body

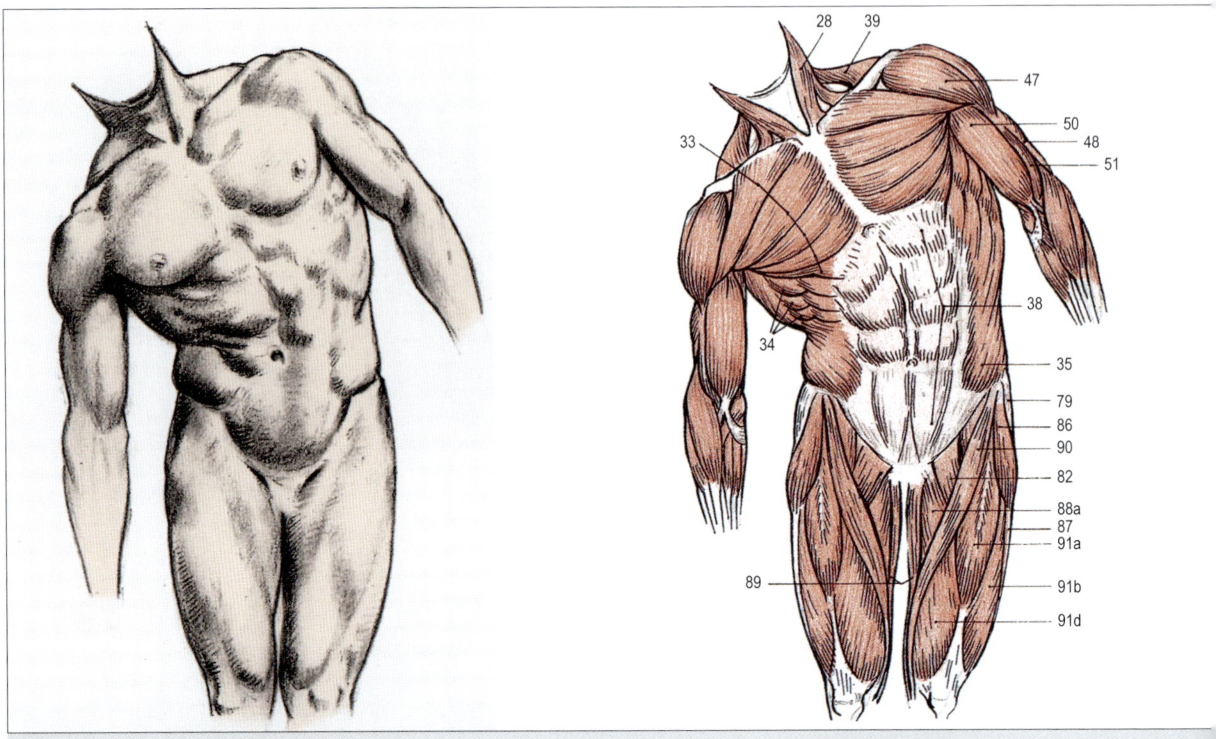

Fig. 90 Basic movement for the lateral inclination of the trunk, showing the active muscle slings (anterior view).

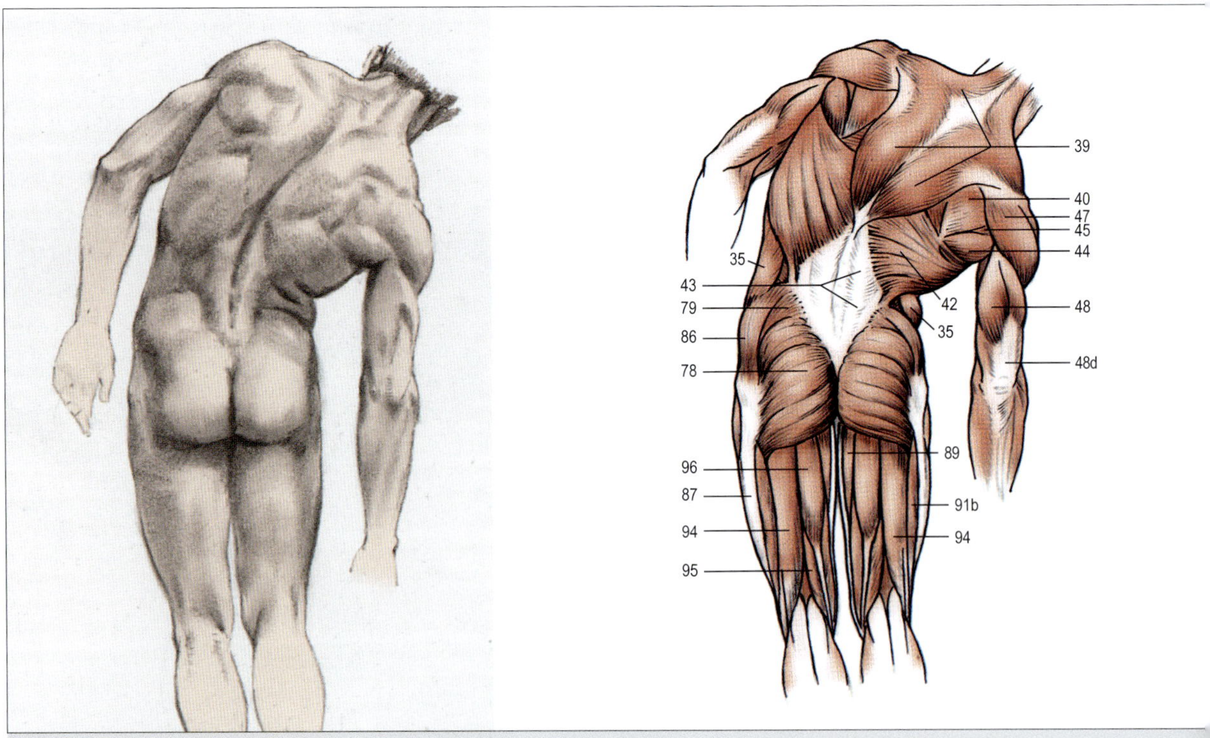

Fig. 91 Basic movement for the lateral inclination of the trunk, showing the active muscle slings (posterior view).

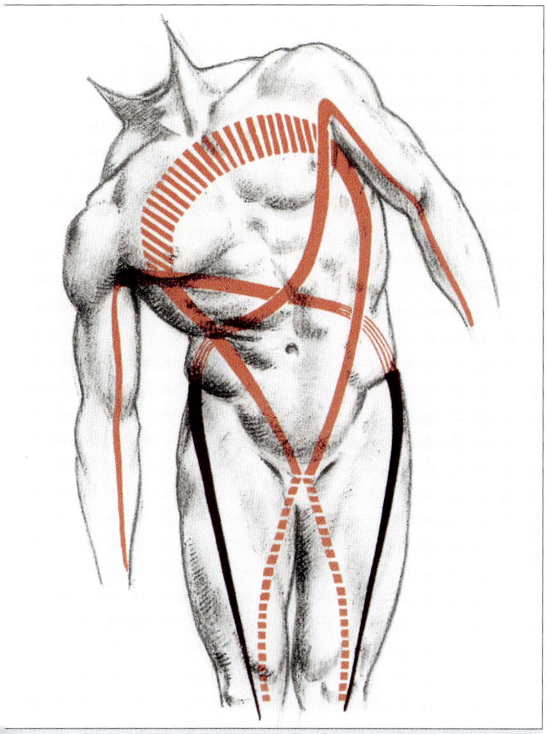

Muscles Fig. 90

- **28** Sternocleido-mastoideus
- **33** Pectoralis major
- **34** Serratur anterior
- **35** Obliquus externus abdominis
- **38** Rectus abdominis
- **39** Trapezius
- **47** Deltoideus
- **48** Triceps brachii
- **50** Biceps brachii
- **51** Brachialis
- **79** Gluteus medius
- **82** Pectineus
- **86** Tensor fasciae latae
- **87** Tractus iliotibialis
- **88a** Adductor longus
- **89** Gracilis
- **90** Sartorius
- **91a** Rectus femoris
- **91b** Vastus lateralis
- **91d** Vastus intermedius

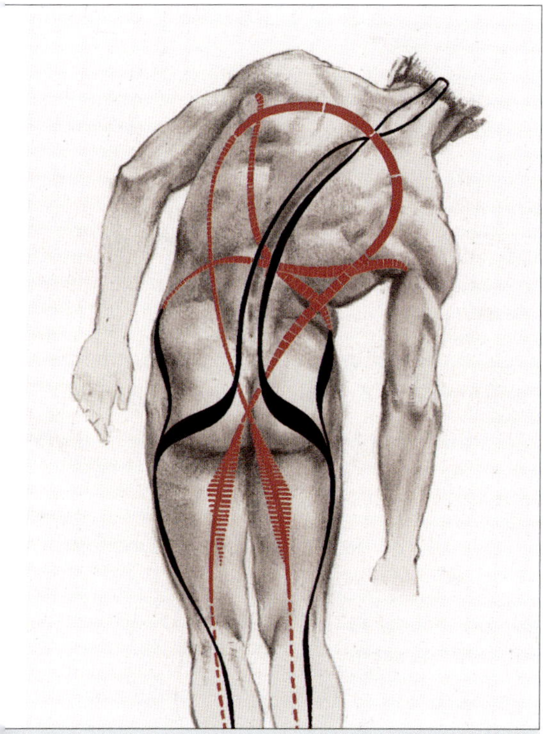

Muscles Fig. 91

- **35** Obliquus externus abdominis
- **39** Trapezius
- **40** Supra- et infraspinatus
- **42** Latissimus dorsi
- **43** Fascia thoracolumbalis
- **44** Teres major
- **45** Teres minor
- **47** Deltoideus
- **48** Triceps brachii
- **48d** Tendon of the arm extensor
- **78** Gluteus maximus
- **79** Gluteus medius
- **87** Tractus iliotibialis
- **91b** Vastus lateralis
- **94** Biceps femoris
- **95** Semimembranosus
- **96** Semitendinosus

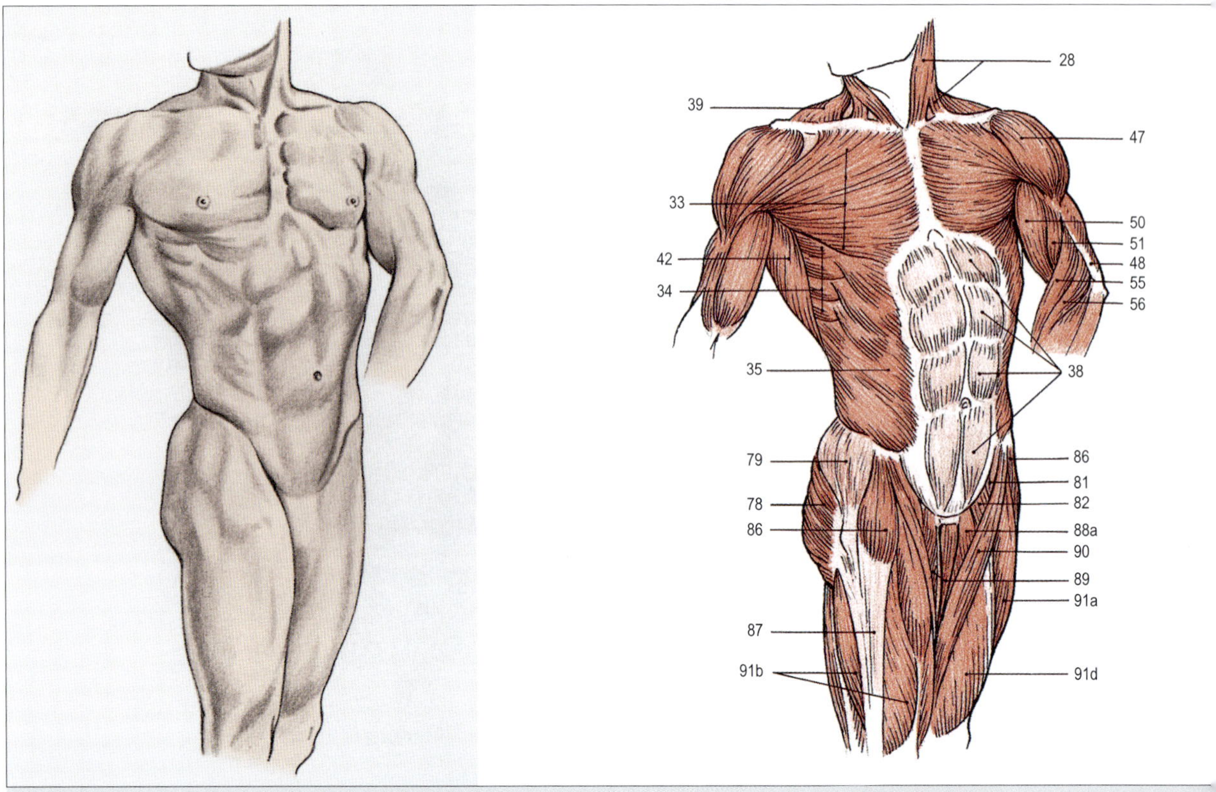

Fig. 92 Basic movement for the rotation, or "wringing" of the trunk, showing the active muscles which rotate the trunk to the right.

Lateral inclincation of the trunk

Some of these combined muscle structures are illustrated in the basic movement of "lateral inclination of the trunk" (fig. 90 and fig. 91) and in the basic movement of "trunk rotation" ("wringing of the trunk") (fig. 92). The **first muscle sling,** which originates together with the rhomboid muscles on the central axial skeleton, continues on over the serratus anterior to the obliquus abdominis externus on the same side of the body, and then crosses over to the other side, namely to the adductors of the thigh, and continues its course over the strands of the short head of the biceps femoris, and on via the head of the fibula, finishing at the fibularis longus and the foot.

The **second muscle sling** has its origin below the lower third of the pectoralis major and continues via the abdominal fascia of the pectoralis major, crosses the body midline, and flows into the fibres of the tendons of the obliquus abdominis internus, which run in the same direction. This combination of muscles comes to an end at the gluteus medius with some strands running into the tensor fascia latae and the tibialis anterior.

Apart from this combination of muscles, the cooperation of two abdominal muscles for the rotation of the trunk should be pointed out. They are actually antagonists, which, in the context of muscle slings responsible for this movement, now become synergists: the **obliquus abdominis internus and the obliquus abdominis externus of the opposite side of the body,** the obliquus abdominis internus drawing its partner towards itself – because of the connection via the rectus sheath and the fibres running in the same direction. As a consequence, the trunk is rotated towards the side of the obliquus abdominis internus (fig. 93 and 94). This example also makes clear that the effectiveness of this kind of cooperation in dynamic sequences of movement is determined both **by the contractile strength of the one muscle and by the degree to which it**

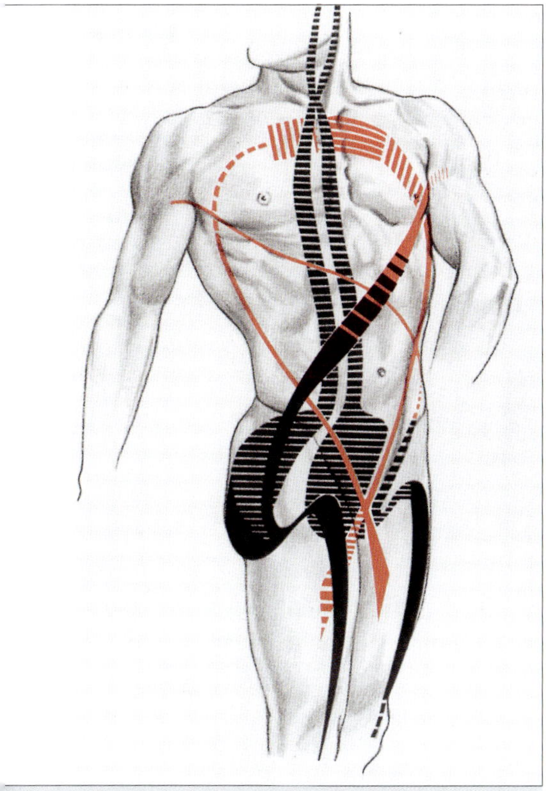

Muscles Fig. 92

- **28** Sternocleido-mastoideus
- **33** Pectoralis major
- **34** Serratus anterior
- **35** Obliquus externus abdominis
- **38** Rectus abdominis
- **39** Trapezius
- **42** Latissimus dorsi
- **47** Deltoideus
- **48** Triceps brachii
- **50** Biceps brachii
- **51** Brachialis
- **55** Brachioradialis
- **56** Extensor carpi radialis longus
- **78** Gluteus maximus
- **79** Gluteus medius
- **81** Iliopsoas
- **82** Pectineus
- **86** Tensor fasciae latae
- **87** Tractus iliotibialis
- **88a** Adductor longus
- **89** Gracilis
- **90** Sartorius
- **91a** Rectus femoris
- **91b** Vastus lateralis
- **91d** Vastus intermedius

partner can be extended, which is a condition of the maintenance of muscle balance.

The fact that this muscle sling is of crucial importance will be shown by considering once more the sudden lifting of the left leg (fig. 95). When the left leg is lifted very high, the following muscle chain – obliquus abdominis externus on the **left** ➔ aponeurosis ➔ obliquus abdominis internus on the **right** – comes into action, so that the left hip joint and, with it, the left leg can be lifted higher

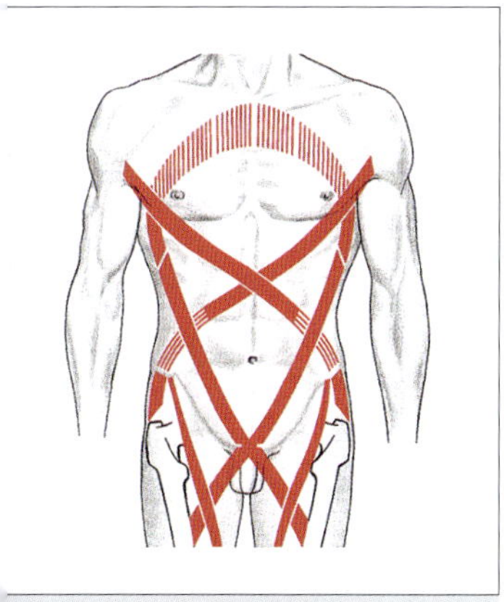

Fig. 93 Schematic illustrations of some muscle slings in which the abdominal muscles are involved.

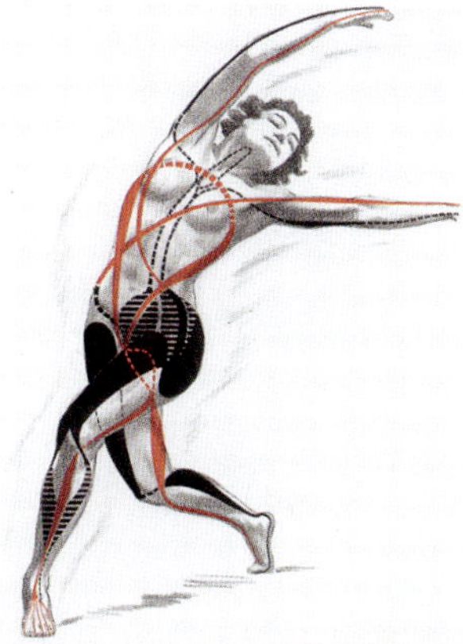

Fig. 94 Muscle slings in lateral inclination and rotation of the trunk in rhythmic gymnastics.

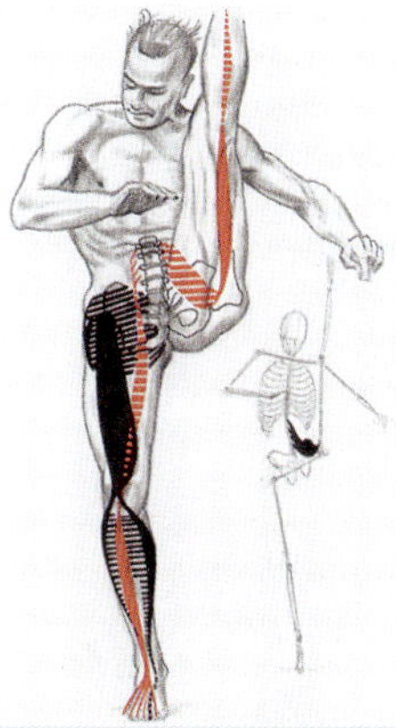

Fig. 95 Muscle slings in sudden lifting of the left leg.

by means of the iliopsoas. This is achieved with the help of the right gluteus medius and minimus.

Finally, the **cooperation of the abdominal muscles with the gluteus maximus** should be mentioned once again. This muscle determines the degree of **pelvic inclination** by its tone or its powerful contraction. A change in pelvic inclination is not possible without the cooperation of the abdominal muscles, which originate partly from the iliac crest and the inguinal ligament, and insert – like the rectus abdominis – into the symphysis.

If the inclination of the pelvis is increased, the abdominal muscles will be stretched, because the lower part of the skeletal frame, in which they are tightly inserted, moves further away from the upper part, the costal arch. The anteriorly inclined pelvis is raised again by the powerful abdominal muscles (and their contraction).

> *"... we are actually able to rock the pelvis on the heads of the femur by the alternating contraction of the abdominal muscles and the gluteus maximus on the one hand, and the iliopsoas on the other. These are movements which, of course, very closely involve the spine, which has to follow every movement of the pelvis, and especially every alteration of pelvic inclination. One can say that the pelvic inclination in a human being is determined by the play and counterplay of all the muscles which originate from the pelvis and run cranially or caudally."* (Hoepke, 1971)

The cooperation of all the muscles mentioned also has a **stabilizing function,** which we have already encountered (fig. 96)

- in wrestling (standing combat)
- in rowing
- in weight-lifting.

This underlines, in an impressive way, **the important role played by the abdominal muscles in dynamic and static sequences of movements,** in the context of large whole-body muscle slings which can be observed very clearly in people who have suffered a loss of function of one of the abdominal muscles as a result of a sports injury, which significantly limits the sequence of movements.

These remarks will make it easier for the reader to understand the following **fast and powerful sequences of movements,** which are characterized, above all, by lateral inclination and rotation of the trunk, and their functionality and beauty.

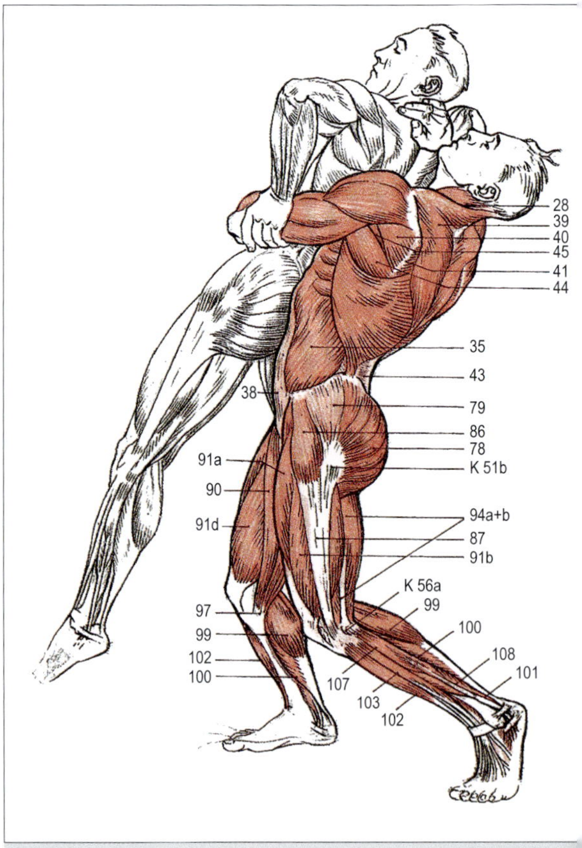

Fig. 96 The stabilizing function of the abdominal muscles in dynamic and static sequences of movements.

Muscles Fig. 96

- **28** Sternocleidomastoideus
- **33** Pectoralis major
- **34** Serratus anterior
- **35** Obliquus externus abdominis
- **38** Rectus abdominis
- **39** Trapezius
- **40** Supra- and infraspinatus
- **41** Rhomboideus major
- **42** Latissimus dorsi
- **43** Fascia thoracolumbalis
- **44** Teres major
- **45** Teres minor
- **47** Deltoideus
- **48** Triceps brachii
- **48d** Tendon of the triceps brachii
- **49** Anconeus
- **50** Biceps brachii
- **50a** Aponeurosis of the biceps brachii
- **51** Brachialis
- **52** Coracobrachialis
- **53** Pronator teres
- **55** Brachioradialis
- **56** Extensor carpi radialis longus
- **57** Extensor carpi radialis brevis
- **58** Extensor carpi ulnaris
- **59** Flexor carpi ulnaris
- **60** Extensor digitorum
- **61** Flexor carpi radialis
- **62** Flexor digitorum superficialis
- **64** Palmaris longus
- **67** Extensor pollicis brevis
- **68** Abductor pollicis longus
- **78** Gluteus maximus
- **79** Gluteus medius
- **86** Tensor fasciae latae
- **87** Tractus iliotibialis
- **88c** Adductor magnus
- **89** Gracilis
- **90** Sartorius
- **91a** Rectus femoris
- **91b** Vastus lateralis
- **91d** Vastus intermedius
- **94** Biceps femoris
- **94a** Biceps femoris, caput longum
- **94b** Biceps femoris, caput breve
- **95** Semimembranosus
- **96** Semitendinosus
- **97** Pes anserinus
- **99** Gastrocnemius
- **100** Soleus
- **101** Tendo calcaneus
- **102** Tibialis anterior
- **103** Extensor digitorum longus
- **104** Extensor digitorum brevis
- **107** Fibularis longus
- **108** Fibularis brevis
- **110** Flexor digitorum longus
- **113** Abductor hallucis

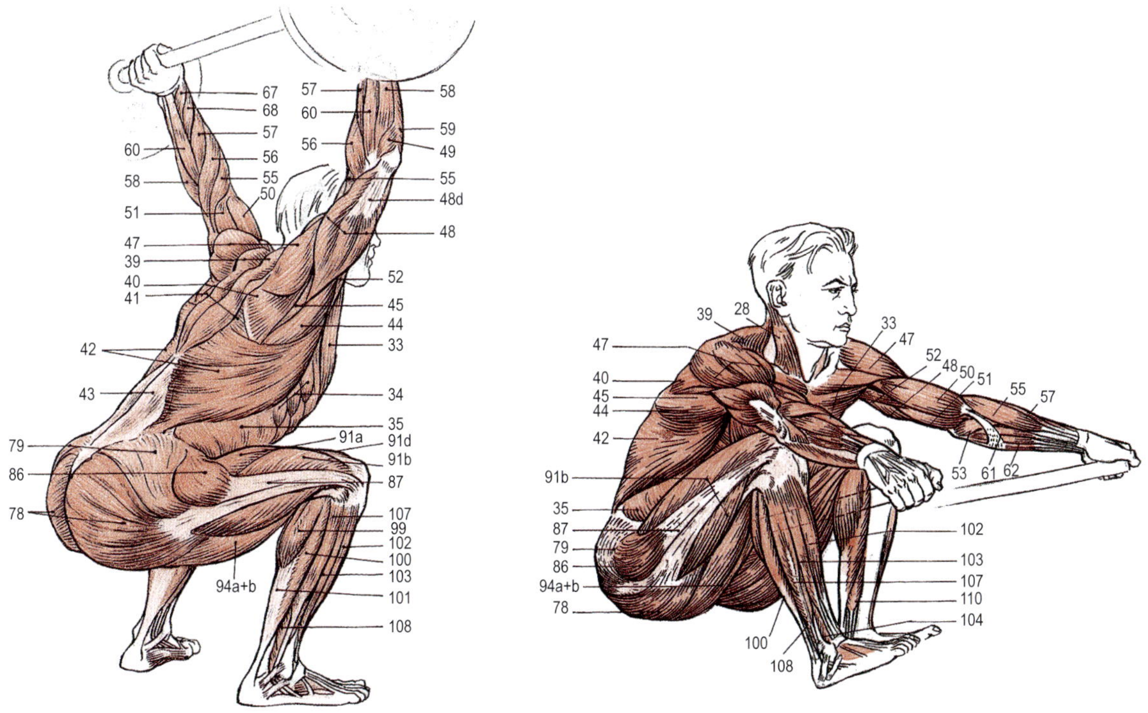

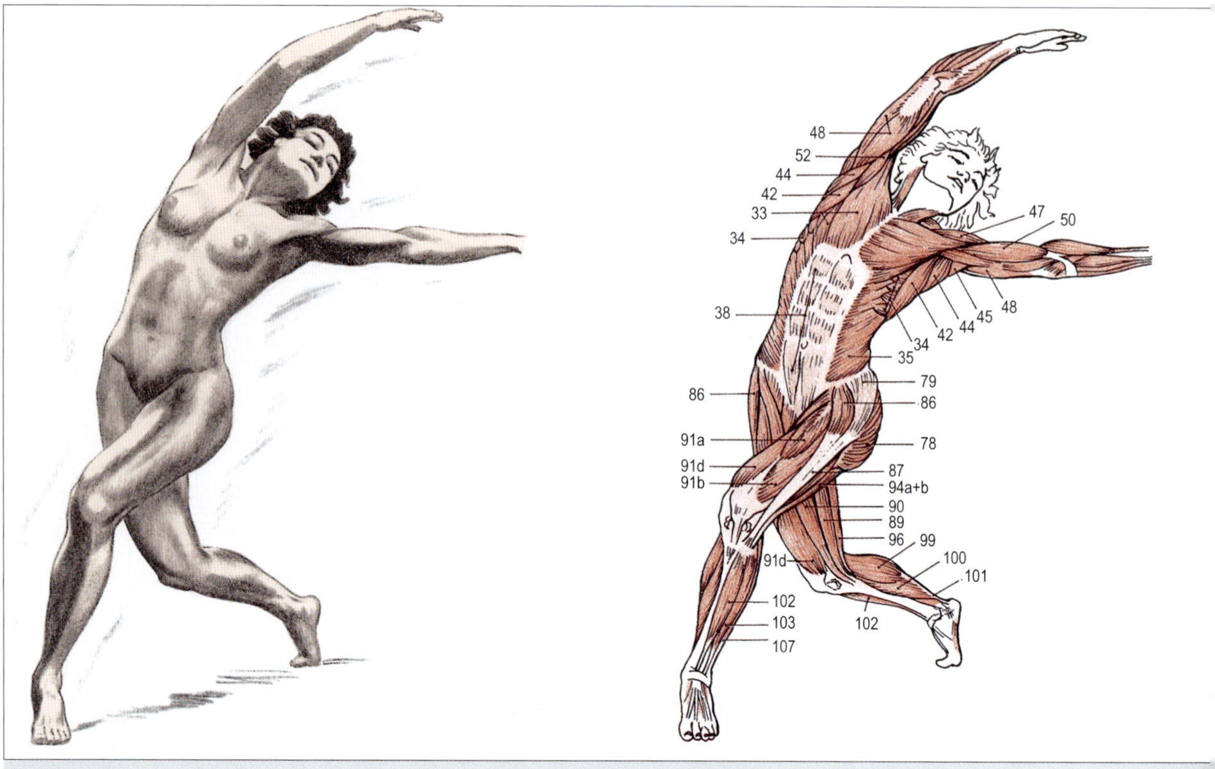

Fig. 97 Muscle slings in lateral inclination and rotation of the trunk in rhythmic gymnastics.

Rhythmic gymnastics

Rhythmic gymnastics (fig. 97) is one of the technical and acrobatic sport disciplines for women, in which handheld equipment (ball, ribbon, club, hoop, rope) is thrown, bounced, and held while rotating it, and swung with great accuracy. This requires the development of superb **coordinative capabilities** and of the vestibular and kinaesthetic system for spacial orientation, and the capability of moving at high rotational speed. The rhythmic gymnast demonstrates clearly how the difficult, novel, stable, aesthetic, fast and powerful movements, in the shoulder joints, and in the clavicular joints (for extreme ante- and retroversion and rotation of the arm) as well as in the hip joints (for extreme abduction, flexion and extension of the leg in jumping) constantly merge into one another, and are thus to be understand as links in a functional chain.

What we learn from this is that there is no movement of the arms or legs which is carried out exclusively at the shoulder or hip joint. **It always requires the whole system.** All the other links in the skeletal and muscle chain ultimately benefit from this because the wide and precise scope of movement which they carry out, can always be attributed to the cooperation and to the coordinated interplay of the shoulder joint and the shoulder girdle muscles or of the muscles of the hip joint and to their sling-like continuation over the whole of the body.

On the other hand, the **specific mobility of the spine and the large joints** in the movement illustrated requires a well-developed stretching capacity, especially of those muscles which tend to shorten their normal length. **Stretching capability** is also an important condition for power training and is a preventative measure to avoid overstraining of the connective and supportive tissue. It is therefore worthwhile including a suitable time in one's preparation for stretching exercises at the beginning and end of each training unit.

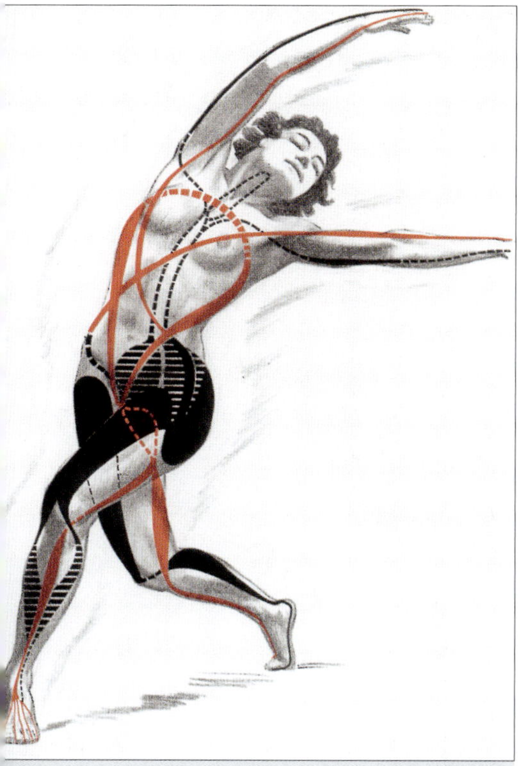

Muscles Fig. 97

33 Pectoralis major
34 Serratus anterior
35 Obliquus externus abdominis
38 Rectus abdominis
42 Latissimus dorsi
44 Teres major
45 Teres minor
47 Deltoideus
48 Triceps brachii
50 Biceps brachii
52 Coracobrachialis
78 Gluteus maximus
79 Gluteus medius
86 Tensor fasciae latae
87 Tractus iliotibialis
89 Gracilis
90 Sartorius
91a Rectus femoris
91b Vastus lateralis
91d Vastus intermedius
94a Biceps femoris, caput longum
94b Biceps femoris, caput breve
96 Semitendinosus
99 Gastrocnemius
100 Soleus
101 Tendo calcaneus
102 Tibialis anterior
103 Extensor digitorum longus
107 Fibularis longus

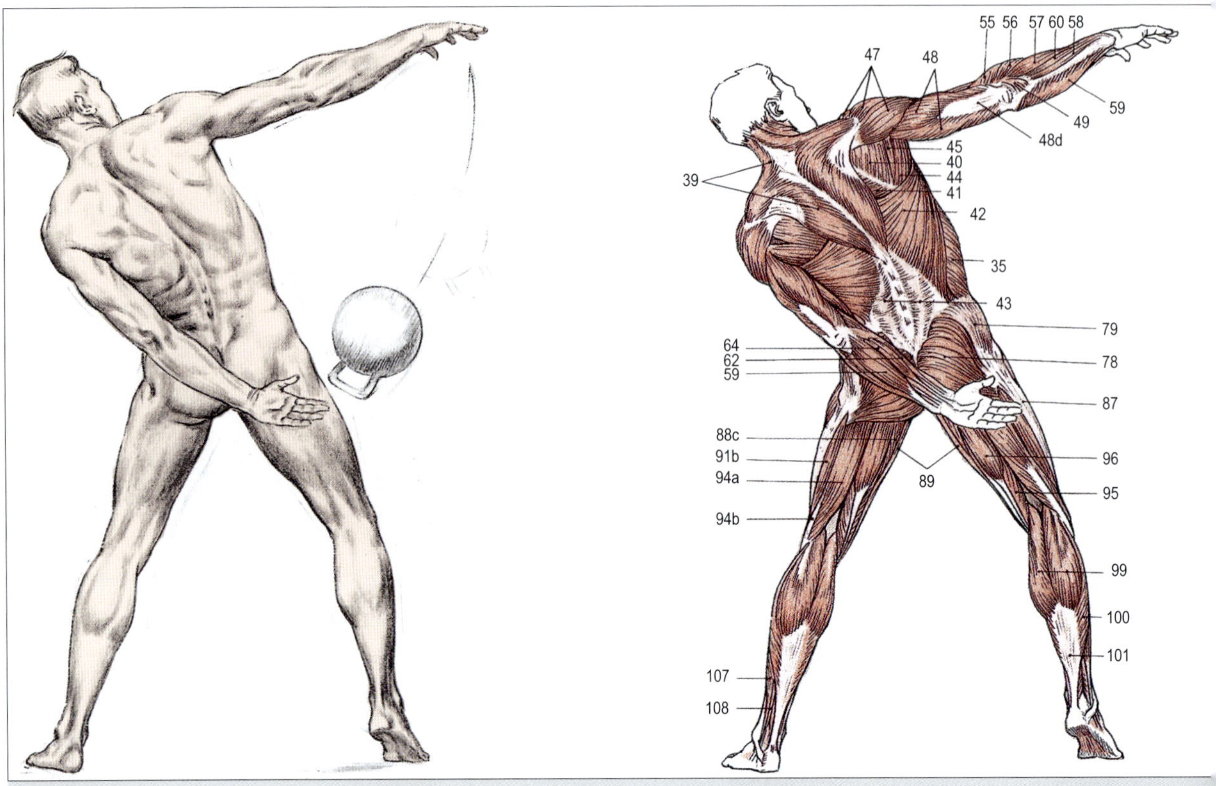

Fig. 98 Muscle slings in lateral inclination and rotation of the trunk, when doing gymnastics with a round weight.

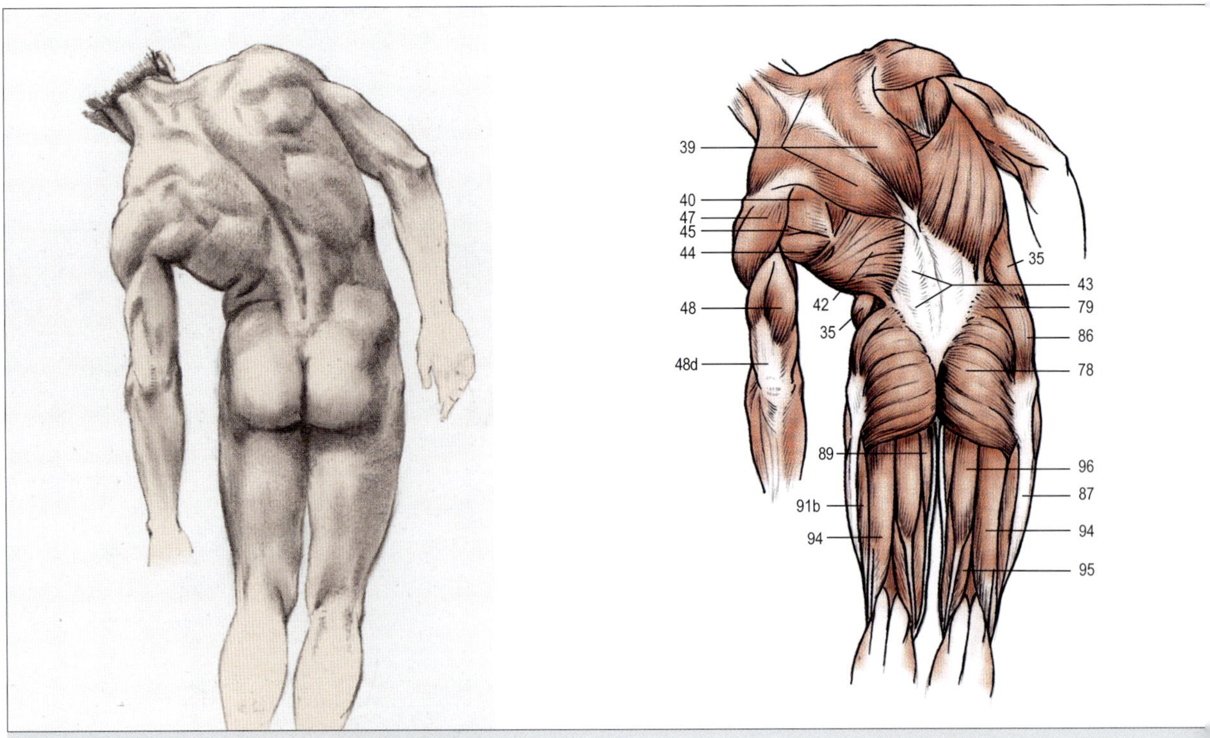

Fig. 99 Basic movement for the lateral inclination of the trunk.

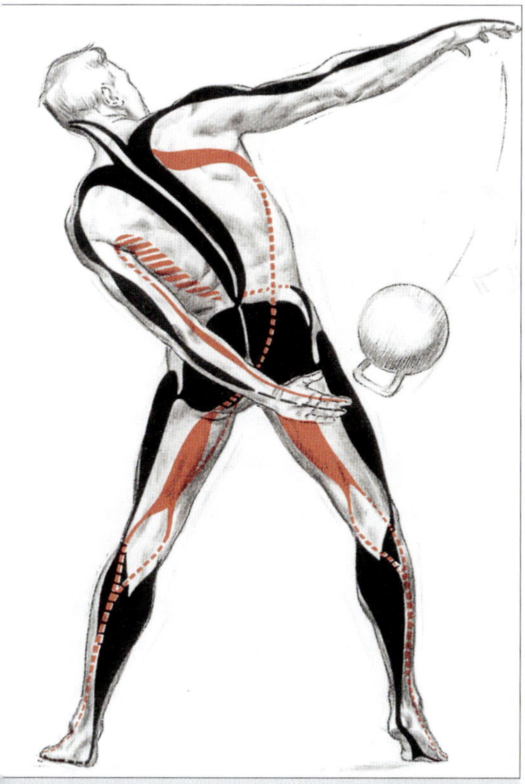

Muscles Fig. 98 and 99

- **35** Obliquus externus abdominis
- **39** Trapezius
- **40** Supra- et infraspinatus
- **41** Rhomboideus major
- **42** Latissimus dorsi
- **43** Fascia thoracolumbalis
- **44** Teres major
- **45** Teres minor
- **47** Deltoideus
- **48** Triceps brachii
- **48d** Tendon of triceps brachii
- **49** Anconeus
- **55** Brachioradialis
- **56** Extensor carpi radialis longus
- **57** Extensor carpi radialis brevis
- **58** Extensor carpi ulnaris
- **59** Flexor carpi ulnaris
- **60** Extensor digitorum
- **62** Flexor digitorum superficialis
- **64** Palmaris longus
- **78** Gluteus maximus
- **79** Gluteus medius
- **87** Tractus iliotibialis
- **88c** Adductor magnus
- **89** Gracilis
- **91b** Vastus lateralis
- **94** Biceps femoris
- **94a** Biceps femoris, caput longum
- **94b** Biceps femoris, caput breve
- **95** Semimembranosus
- **96** Semitendinosus
- **99** Gastrocnemius
- **100** Soleus
- **101** Tendo calcaneus
- **107** Fibularis longus
- **108** Fibularis brevis

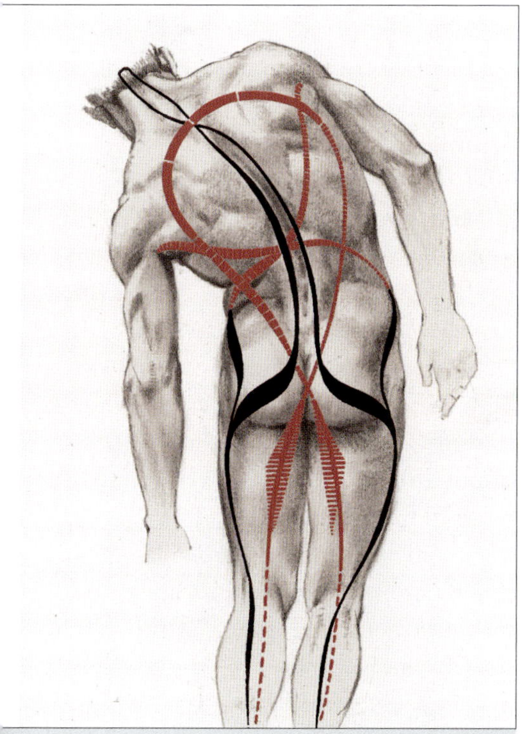

Gymnastics with round weights

In women's gymnastics it is mainly clubs, hoops, rubber or plastic balls, ropes, rods, flags or ribbons which are used as instruments. In men's gymnastics medicine balls, shots or round weights are used. They have the effect of increasing muscle strength and shaping the body because of their weight (10–12 kg).

The illustrations (fig. 98 and 99) give us an opportunity to revise what we have learned so far about the mode of operation of muscle slings in lateral inclination and rotation of the trunk, before we turn to the next sequences of movements.

The central role of the knee joint in many sports disciplines

The knee joint is the largest joint of the human motor system with the strongest ligaments, the most complicated mechanics and the highest incidence of injuries and inappropriate load. In comparison with other joints it is characterized by its **opposing functions:**

- when the leg is extended it has a stable supporting and weight-bearing function
- when the leg is flexed it guarantees its mobility.

The knee joint, which is important for statics and dynamics, is a functional rotary hinge joint (trocho-ginglymus). It enables the leg to bend and extend around a frontal axis and an outward rotation of 15° around a vertical axis in the last 20° before complete extension of the lower leg (final rotation). This occurs in three functionally closely cooperating parts of the joint consisting of

- the convex surfaces of the joint of both femoral epicondyles
- the almost even joint surfaces of the tibial epicondyles and
- the posterior surface of the patella.

All of these make up the **proximal and distal femoro-tibial** and **femoro-patellar joint.**

As a result of this, the first two joint surfaces differ in shape and show an incongruence in the radius of curvature, so that they are in contact only in a punctuate or linear manner, particularly when the leg is flexed. This **incongruence is compensated** for by a 3–4 mm thick hyaline cartilage coating of the joint to absorb the effects of shock and pressure which act upon the knee joint when walking, landing after jumping and lifting a heavy weight. The same effect is achieved by the c-shaped and cuneiform (when seen from above and from the side) fibrocartilaginous discs, the **medial and lateral meniscus** (fig. 100).

It should be emphasized that the medial, crescent-shaped meniscus is in close contact, via the articular capsule, with the medial collateral ligament. The lateral, spherical meniscus is in close contact only with the articular capsule, but not with the lateral collateral ligament. This is why dynamic tensile loads on these ligaments, especially in football and alpine ski sports (see below) are transferred to the menisci and can cause injury, especially to the medial meniscus.

When the knee joint is moved, the somewhat mobile **menisci are shifted slightly backwards** by 1 cm by the condyles of the femur against the plane of the tibial head when the leg is flexed, and shifted forwards when the leg is extended (fig. 101). When the lower leg is rotated outwards, the lateral meniscus is shifted forwards, the medial meniscus is drawn backwards, and vice versa when rotated inwards. The torsion and hinge movements of the bended knee must therefore be complemented by sliding movements. Hence the menisci bear not only part of the axial weight on the knee joint, but also function as mobile joint sockets.

Because the medial and lateral collateral ligaments are relaxed in the flexed labile position of the knee joint, the menisci and the cruciate ligaments constitute a **functional unity,** which secures the necessary stability of the knee joint when it is extended, flexed and rotated outwardly and inwardly.

The knee joint is held in position and secured, not by bones (like the elbow joint), not primarily by muscles (like the shoulder joint), but above all by strong ligaments, namely the **collateral and cruciate ligaments.**

The main function of the tibial and fibular collateral ligaments (fig. 100–103) is to stabilize the weight-supporting leg (when it is extended), particularly by shifting the centre of gravity of the body anteriorly to the transverse axis of the hip joint, and, by means of their tension, to stabilize the weight-bearing column. The cruciate ligaments (fig. 100 and 102), on the other hand, which are situated within this joint, constrain a maximal forward and backward movement of the joint surfaces, when the leg is in a flexed and vulnerable, labile position in which the collateral ligaments are relaxed and thus unable to function. Thanks to the stability of their strong, intersecting fibre strands, they limit the rotary movements of the lower leg (fig. 102): when the internal rotation of the lower leg is more pronounced, the cruciate ligaments wind around

Front of the joint capsule with the quadriceps muscle severed and the patella folded downwards;

External surface of the femoral joint and synovial fold have been removed to give a better view of the menisci and the transversal ligament.

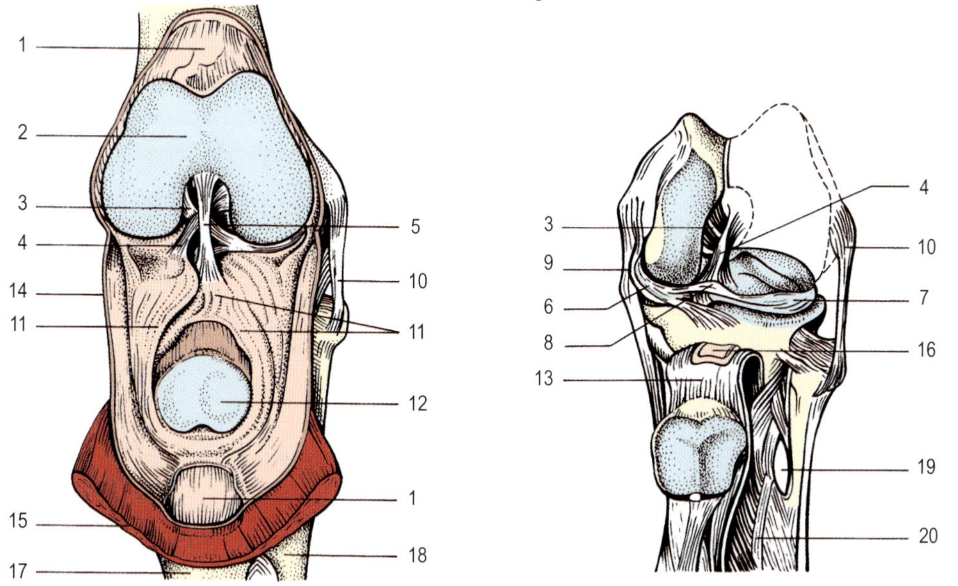

1 Bursa above the patella (Bursa suprapatellaris)
2 Furrow between the surfaces of the femoral joint (Facies patellaris)
3 Posterior cruciate ligament (Lig. cruciatum posterius)
4 Anterior cruciate ligament (Lig. cruciatum anterius)
5 Synovial fold (Plica synovialis infrapatellaris)
6 Medial meniscus
7 Lateral meniscus
8 transversal ligament (Lig. transversum genus)
9 Medial (tibial) collateral ligament (Lig. collaterale tibiale)
10 Fibular (lateral) collateral ligament (Lig. collaterale fibulare)
11 Wing folds (Plicae alares)
12 Patella (Patella)
13 Patellar ligament (Lig. patellae)
14 Articular capsule (section edge) (Capsula articularis)
15 Section edge of the quadriceps femoris
16 Bursa underneath the patella (Bursa infrapatellaris)
17 Tibia (Tibia)
18 Fibula (Fibula)
19 Opening for the anterior tibial artery (A. tibialis anterior)
20 Interosseous membrane of the lower leg (Membrana interossea cruris)

Fig. 100 Left knee joint (anterior view).

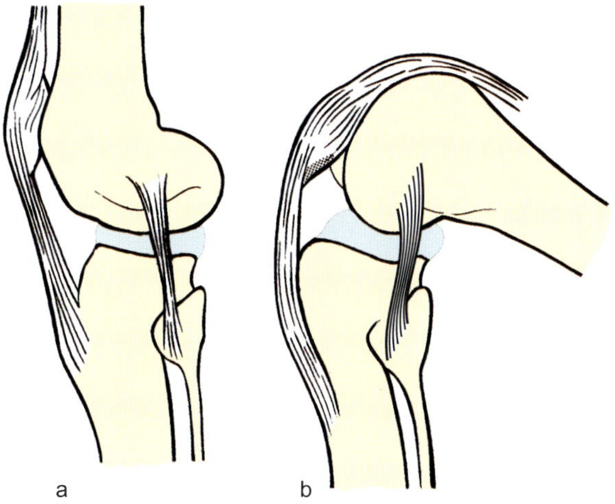

Fig. 101 Flexion of the knee joint.
Final phase: the menisco-femoral joint gliding 1 cm posteriorly. Relaxation of the collateral fibular ligament.

each other and then unwind again when the lower leg is in external rotation.

This specific structure of the knee joint and its specific constituents (menisci, collateral and cruciate ligaments) explain **why certain types of sport,** in which the rotation of the flexed knee joint is particularly pronounced (such as in football, handball, ski slalom, ice hockey and riding), **are prone to an increased risk of injury to the menisci as well as to the connected ligament strands:**

- specific constellations in football such as "landing on one leg after jumping towards the ball",
- rapid changes of direction such as "sudden external rotation in the flexed knee joint when at the same time the foot is fixed by the boot studs in the pitch and sudden breaking or acceleration when running",

which cause a jerky, drawer-like sliding of the tibia against the fibula, bring about an external rotation or valgus position. This endangers the anterior cruciate ligament because its muscular partners – the ischiocrural muscles on the back of the thighs – are too weak in this position to secure the surface of the tibia and with it the anterior cruciate ligament. In football, where the knee joint is particularly vulnerable, the **anterior cruciate ligament can rupture.** This occurs in women's football, in two thirds of the cases without any contact with an opponent (Faude et al. 2005), 7–8 times more frequently than in men's football (Becker et al. 2005,Tittel 2012).

In what way does the **sequence of movement specific to football in women differ from that in men?** In women the angle of the flexed knee is only 17° when they land after jumping towards the ball, but in men it comes to 33°. This means that women complete their jump in a more upright position with greater impact and in more pronounced valgus position, which leads to greater anterior shearing forces and these put a lot of strain on the anterior cruciate ligament and the joint cartilage.

Because of the broader pelvis and the associated smaller angle between the neck and the shaft of the femur (below 128°) as well as the larger Q-angle in women (fig. 103) the on-average shorter thighs in women converge towards the knee joint to a greater extent than in men and form a physiological knock-kneed position (genu valgum). As a result of this the quadriceps femoris is stretched much further and this means greater risk of injury for the anterior cruciate ligament.

For this reason it is necessary to consider prevention and to pay **more attention to the muscles involved** (which co-operate in a muscle sling) and to specific training to achieve a stable ligamental system and postural regulation. This applies especially to footballers (see fig. 104 and 105) and their general and specific abilities, especially their acceleration capability, kicking speed, agility and jumping power, as well as the contractile force and ability to relax the muscles just mentioned.

Muscular imbalance makes it necessary, to include, as mentioned, in training special jumping and strengthening elements in order to secure the functional stability of the knee joint. These should be combined with balance exercises, in order to **increase the activity of the ischiocrural muscles,** which have a tendency to shorten their length and are a "problem area" in football (and in alpine ski sports).

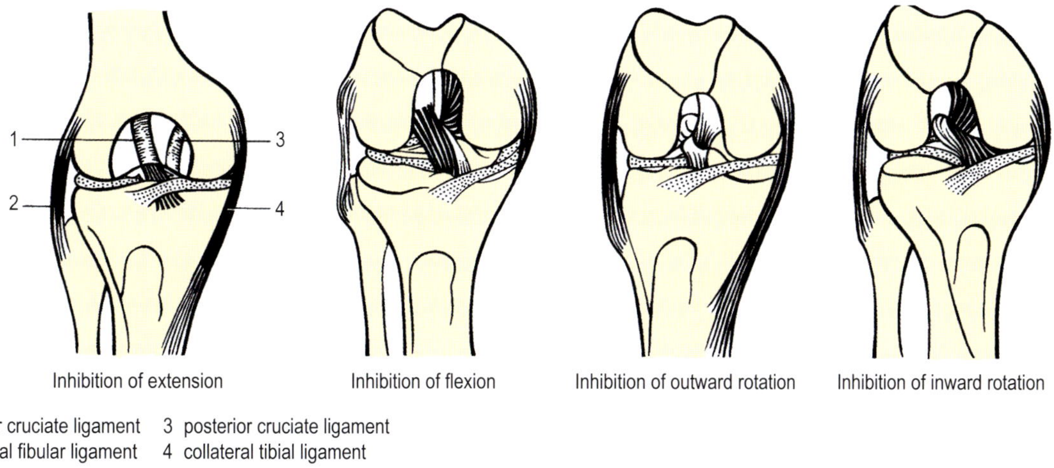

Fig. 102 Functional partnership of cruciate and collateral ligaments when the knee joint is extended, flexed and rotated internally and externally. The tense ligamental strands are darker, the relaxed ones are lighter.

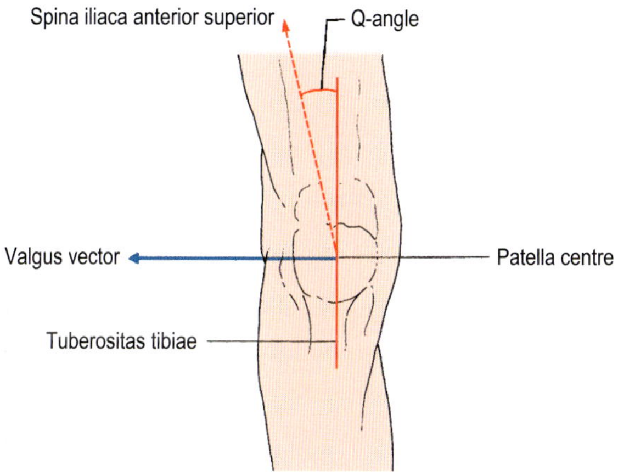

Fig. 103 The so-called Q-angle is the angle between the vertical axis of the leg and the direction of power exerted by the quadriceps femoris. In women it is 20° and in men 12°, and it increarses the genu valgum.

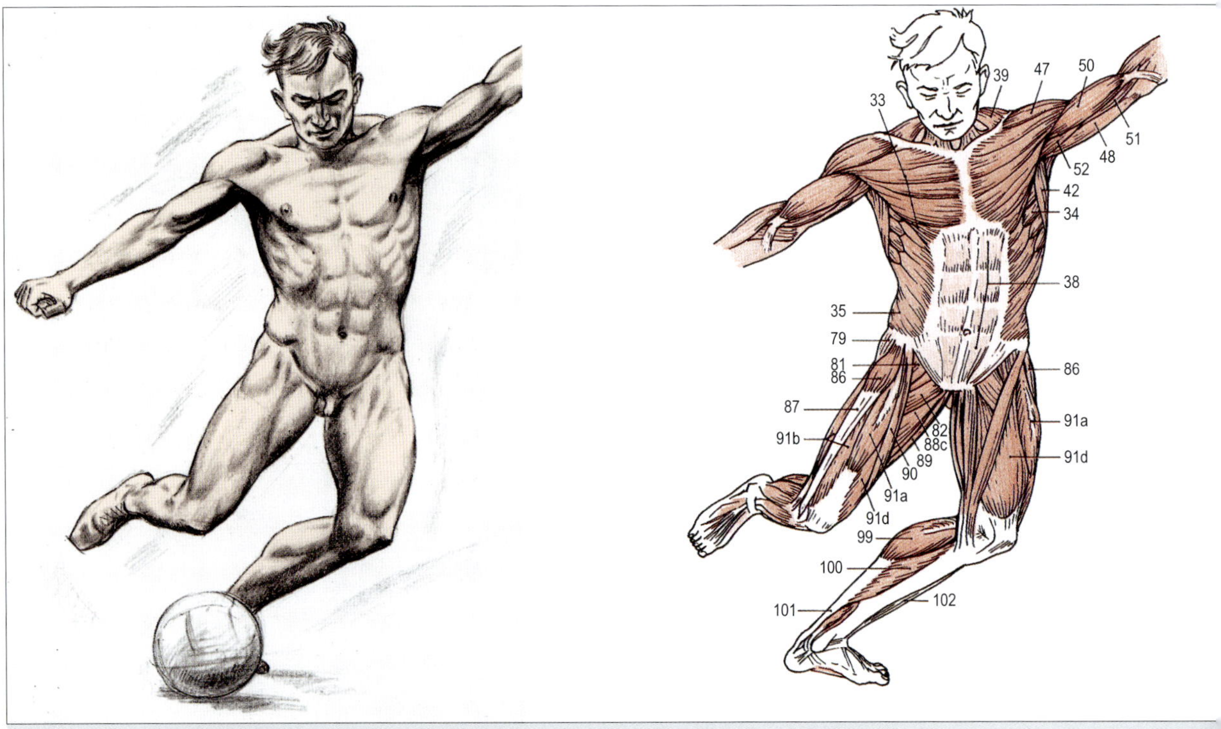

Fig. 104 Muscle slings in lateral inclination and rotation of the trunk to pass the ball.

Football player (crossing the ball)

When a footballer crosses the ball (fig. 104), **the great strain caused by pressure, traction and torsion on the knee joint of the flexed supporting leg** is very obvious. The strain must be absorbed by the muscles and ligaments in order to maintain the body equilibrium. This adjustment of body posture by the supporting leg ("regulation of posture") is important since many techniques in football (shooting and passing the ball) are carried out standing on one leg.

When analyzing the movement of the footballer for crosses, and particularly for shots at goal (fig. 105), it is necessary once more to pay attention first of all to the hip joint, which is brought forward noticeably in order to facilitate the **"preparatory movement"** of the responsible leg muscles. We can also see this in various throwing disciplines (fig. 107–111). The pre-stretched muscles are now able to carry out their work with remarkable power and with the help of the long extensor muscle sling, which runs over the whole body.

This applies to the following **synergists** and – during contact with the ball – also **antagonists** (in brackets):

- for the intensive flexion of the hip joint, the iliopsoas (and gluteus maximus),
- for the explosive extension of the knee joint, the strong quadriceps femoris (and the substantially weaker ischiocrural muscles: biceps femoris, semitendinosus and semimembranosus), as well as
- for the plantar flexion of the upper ankle joint the tibialis anterior (and the gastrocnemius).

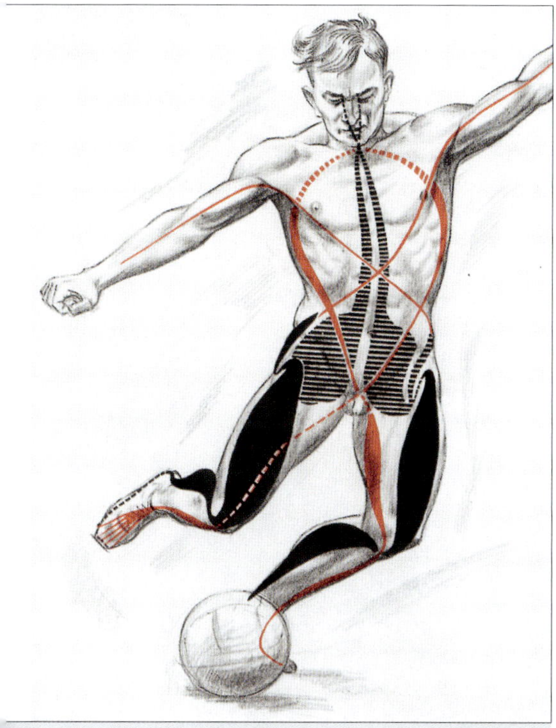

Muscles Fig. 104

33 Pectoralis major
34 Serratus anterior
35 Obliquus externus abdominis
38 Rectus abdominis
39 Trapezius
42 Latissimus dorsi
47 Deltoideus
48 Triceps brachii
50 Biceps brachii
51 Brachialis
52 Coracobrachialis
79 Gluteus medius
81 Iliopsoas
82 Pectineus
86 Tensor fasciae latae
87 Tractus iliotibialis
88c Adductor magnus
89 Gracilis
90 Sartorius
91a Rectus femoris
91b Vastus lateralis
91d Vastus intermedius
99 Gastrocnemius
100 Soleus
101 Tendo calcaneus
102 Tibialis anterior

This functional cooperation requires marked **"muscular balance"** and regular versatile and well-coordinated physical activity, in other words a **good balance between the synergists and antagonists** mentioned above. The discrepancy between the well-trained leg muscles and the often insufficiently trained abdominal and spinal muscles can be caused by the following factors:

- physical inactivity,
- permanent one-sided strain in everyday life and in power training,
- asymmetrical (imbalanced) sport disciplines such as tennis, squash, badminton, fencing,
- the insufficient relaxation and stretch capabilities
- finally individual factors such as age, sex, body-height and -weight.

This interference with the cooperating muscles (**"muscular dys- or imbalance"**) has in many cases also negative consequences for the functions of the joints (**"arthro-muscular dysbalance"**). This may lead to injuries or strain applied incorrectly in various competitive sports. This can cause muscle strain, chronic insertion tendinopathy and cartilage damage. For this reason the first priority should be to achieve and to secure as far as possible the stability of the relationship between muscles and joints.

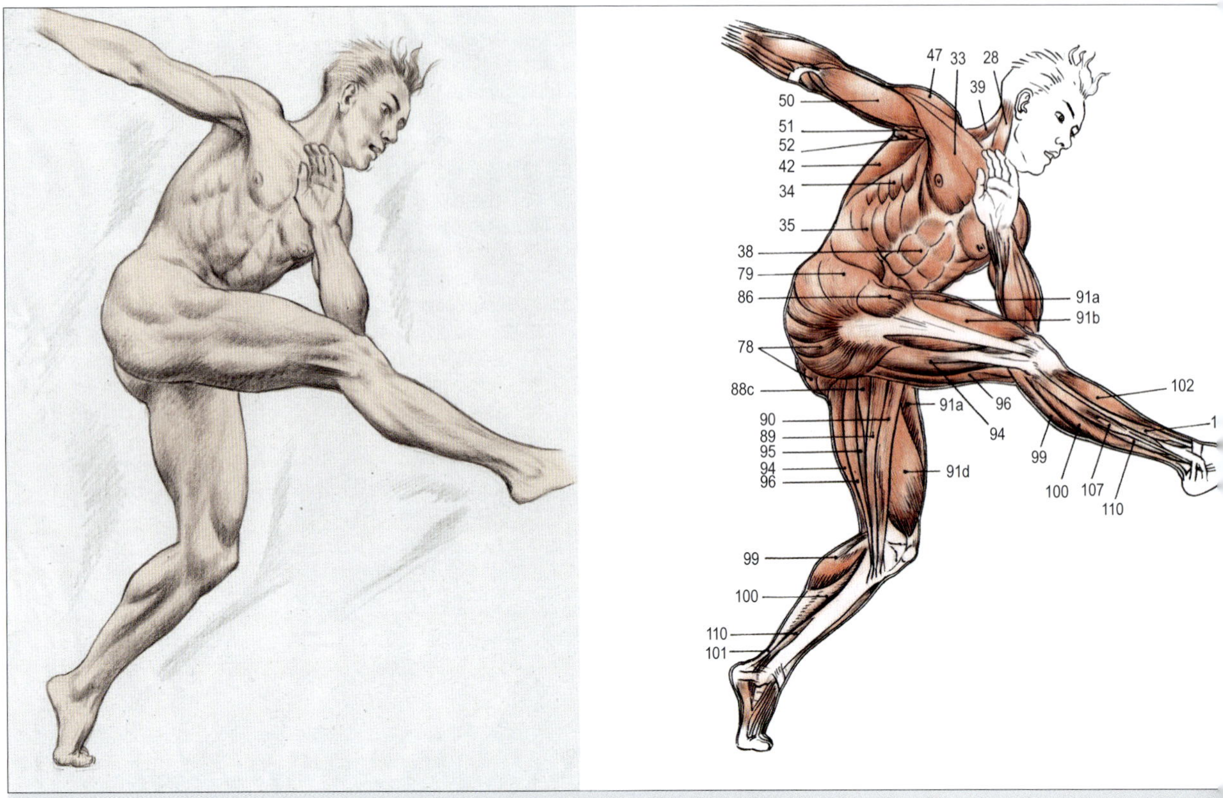

Fig. 105 Muscle slings in anterior inclination of the trunk in a footballer kicking the ball in a volley.

Football player (volleying the ball)

In the second illustration (fig. 105) the rotated upper body of the player is inclined slightly forwards over the ball in order to keep the ball low when kicking it. There are **two important factors for a powerful shot:**

- the interplay of the quadriceps femoris, which is partly doubly feathered and thus very powerful, weighing on average 2 kg with a physiological cross-section of 185 cm^2 with the much weaker ischiocrural muscles, the largest cross-section of which is only 51 cm^2 and
- the interplay of the powerful quadriceps femoris, depending on the specific sport in question, with the abdominal and deep dorsal muscles, which are sometimes weak.

Fig. 106 summarizes the powerful actions of the leg muscles of a footballer kicking a ball. The shared and timed activity of the synergists and the antagonists can be seen very clearly.

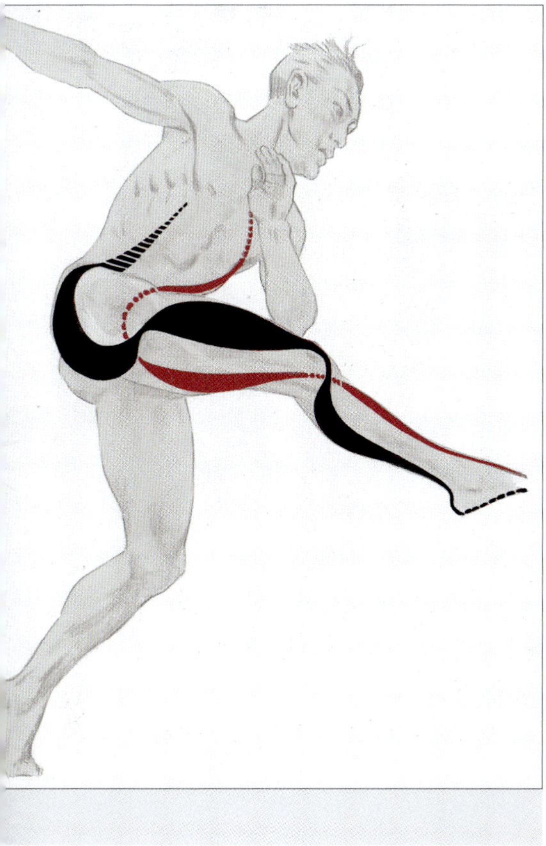

Muscles Fig. 105

28 Sternocleidomastoideus
33 Pectoralis major
34 Serratus anterior
35 Obliquus externus abdominis
38 Rectus abdominis
39 Trapezius
42 Latissimus dorsi
47 Deltoideus
50 Biceps brachii
51 Brachialis
52 Coracobrachialis
78 Gluteus maximus
79 Gluteus medius
86 Tensor fasciae latae
87 Tractus iliotibialis
88c Adductor magnus
89 Gracilis
90 Sartorius
91a Rectus femoris
91b Vastus lateralis
91d Vastus intermedius
94 Biceps femoris
95 Semimembranosus
96 Semitendinosus
99 Gastrocnemius
100 Soleus
101 Tendo calcaneus
102 Tibialis anterior
103 Extensor digitorum longus
107 Fibularis longus
110 Flexor digitorum longus

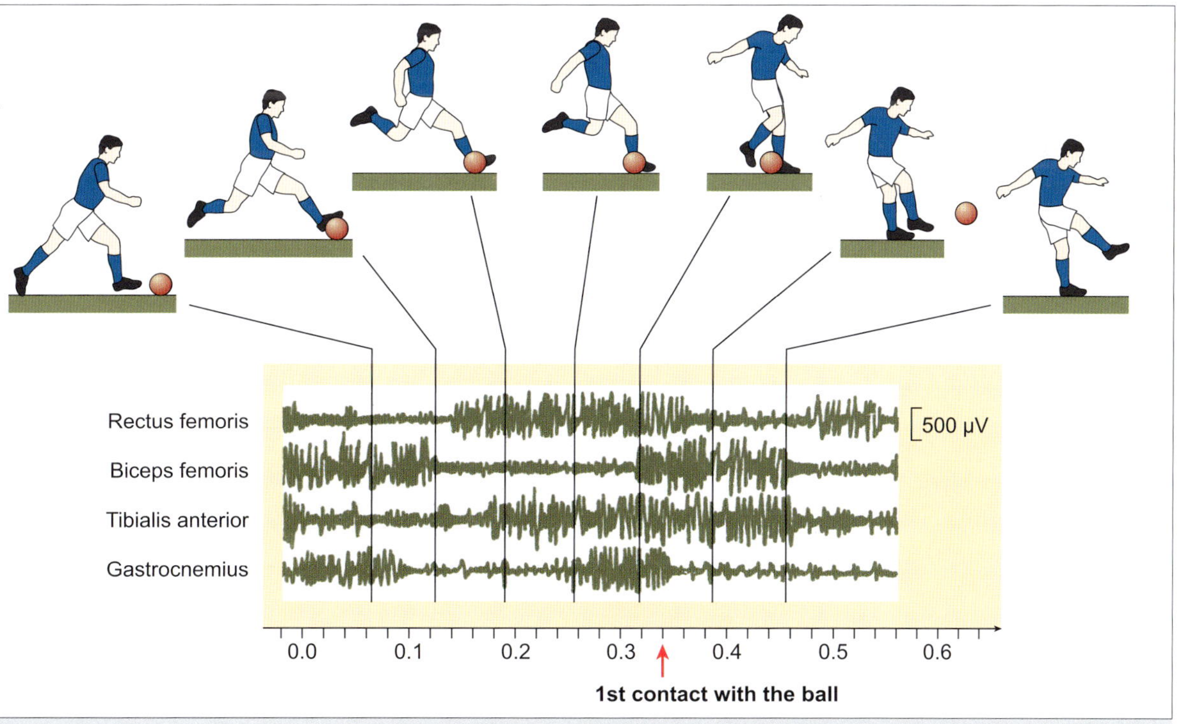

Fig. 106 Bioelectrical activity of the leg muscles of a footballer kicking the ball. The following synergists and antagonists which have already been shown and explained in fig. 105 were tested: rectus femoris, biceps femoris, tibialis anterior and gastrocnemius. The arrow marks the moment of the player's first and powerful contact with the ball.

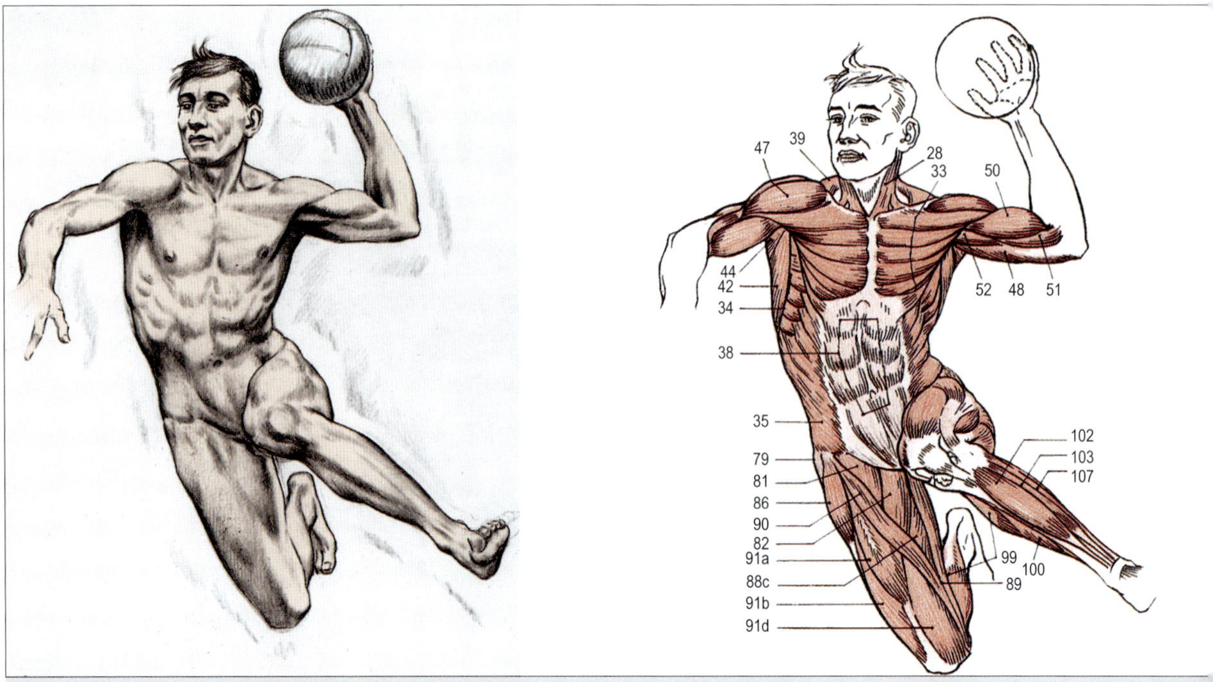

Fig. 107 Muscle slings in lateral inclination and rotation of the trunk in a handball player in a jump shot.

Handball player (jump shot)

The distinctive feature of indoor handball are intermittent stresses, such as frequent changes of sprint, stopping and jumping movements. This sport is characterized by a very dynamic fast and explosive style with (frequently aggressive) physical confrontations and tough encounters between two players, who have psychological and technical competitive stability, a readiness to take risks and tactical discipline, as well as by the increasing deployment of players with a favourable physical constitution.

From time to time there are violent contacts between the players. The jumps and the falls, especially from outside positions into the circle require some preventive measures such as **gum shields** (as in boxing), **jock straps and soft-foam protectors** for the elbow and knee joints, in order to avoid serious injury or chronic stress on the synovial bursae.

For this reason it is not surprising that in this spor discipline players predominate who are notec for their great physical capabilities such as **speec** (speed in sprinting, moving and reacting), **speec in unleashing power** (power in jumping anc throwing) and general as well as specific **enduranc** (endurance in sprinting and fast movements) anc for their well-developed coordinative capabilities which are not least a pre-condition for precise per formance in passing the ball and throwing the bal at the goal.

These performance-determining factors, which in clude an above-average height (190–195 cm fo point guards, 188–190 cm for goal keepers anc 185 cm for pevot players) which increases the leve hold for throwing, are mirrored in the powerfu jump throw of a handball player (fig. 107). Th muscle slings over the whole body can be clearl seen in this very frequent and at the same time ver

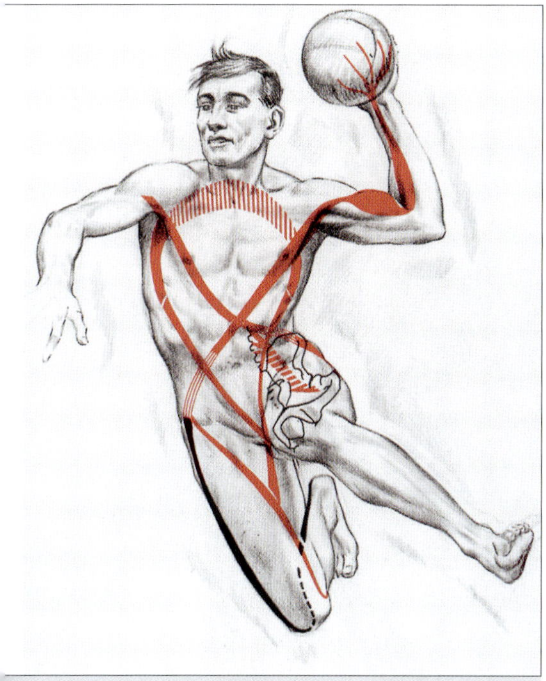

Muscles Fig. 107

28	Sternocleidomastoideus	**81**	Iliopsoas
33	Pectoralis major	**82**	Pectineus
34	Serratus anterior	**86**	Tensor fasciae latae
35	Obliquus externus abdominis	**88c**	Adductor magnus
38	Rectus abdominis	**89**	Gracilis
39	Trapezius	**90**	Sartorius
42	Latissimus dorsi	**91a**	Rectus femoris
44	Teres major	**91b**	Vastus lateralis
47	Deltoideus	**91d**	Vastus intermedius
48	Triceps brachii	**99**	Gastrocnemius
50	Biceps brachii	**100**	Soleus
51	Brachialis	**102**	Tibialis anterior
52	Coracobrachialis	**103**	Extensor digitorum longus
79	Gluteus medius	**107**	Fibularis longus

ffective action of throwing the ball at the goal, which is preceded by an extensive pre-stretching of he muscles involved in throwing (brought about y a posterior rotation of the trunk in the sense of winding-up movement). They are the precondition for jumping power and force of the throw nd this underlines once again the fact that the novement – especially the powerful movement of he throwing arm at the shoulder joint – always equires **the whole system.**

his can be shown with a specific example. In an xplosive jump shot with an intensive rotation and ateral flexion of the trunk, an indoor handball layer suffered, without having been attacked by n opponent, an accident after only three mintes. This was obviously the result of the muscles ot being adapted to stress (perhaps insufficiently varmed-up). A clearly palpable **disruption of the erratus anterior** very close to its functional connection with the **obliquus abdominis externus** was diagnosed. On the 5th day of the healing process with conservative treatment the player said: "I tried to throw the ball very carefully and gently, but I was unable to do this. I don't understand this because my shoulder joint as well as shoulder girdle muscles are as powerful as usual. Why did this happen?"

The answer is obvious and will come as no surprise to the readers of this book: **"The power of a muscle sling will be determined exclusively by the weakest limb in the chain".** For this reason more attention should always be paid to strengthening the whole of the body and to coordination, to an exact technical ability to catch the ball as well as to fall or roll correctly, and to jumping exercises, including the most essential preventive measures, such as proper warming-up prior to sport activities at a very early stage.

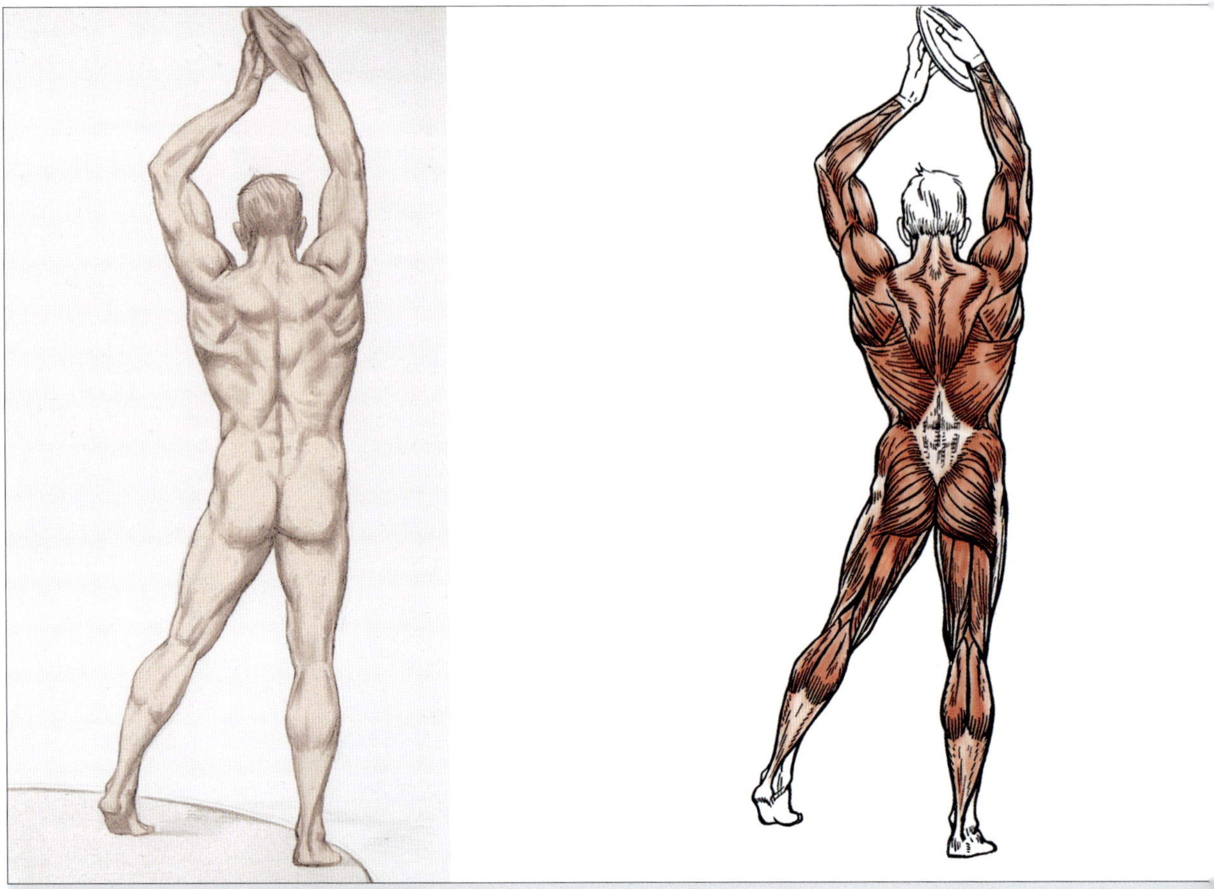

Fig. 108a Muscle slings in a discus thrower in the starting position (prestretching).
After having discussed many muscle slings, the reader should now mark the muscles in the muslce illustration which work together in the muscle slings on the right. (Resolution see http://url9.de/Wzy)

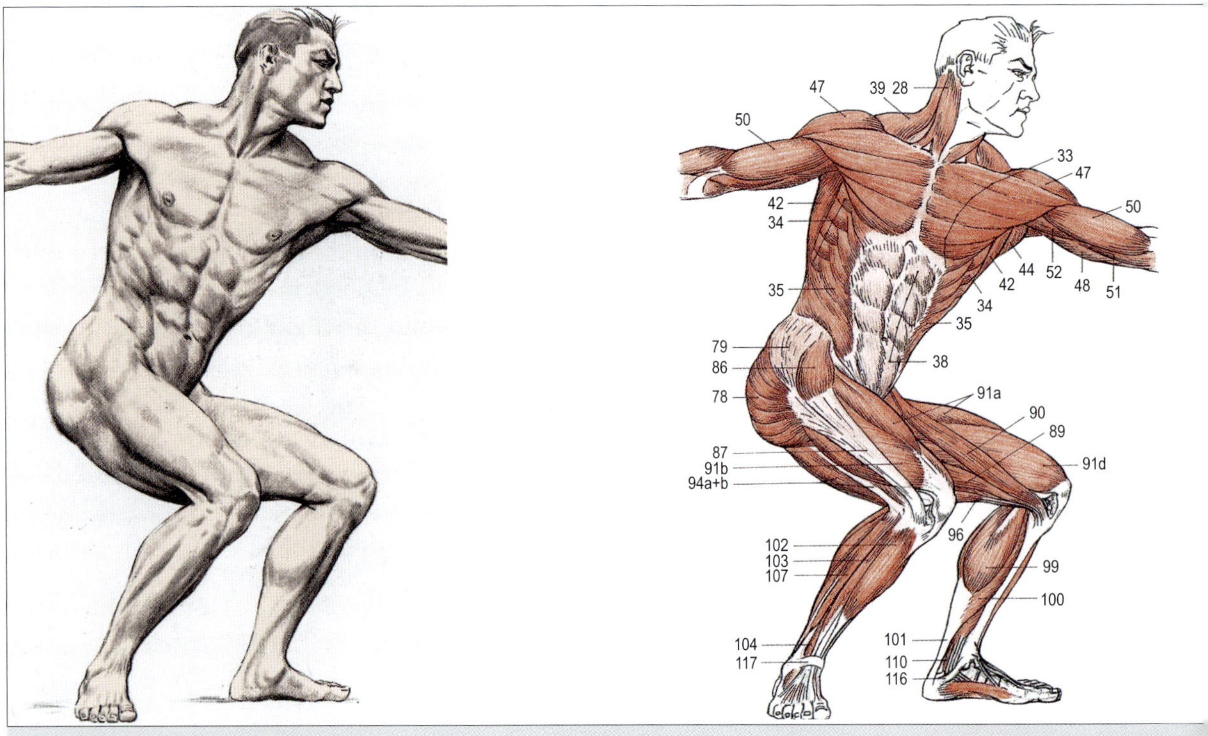

Fig. 108b Muscle slings for torsion ("wringing") of the trunk in a discus thrower.

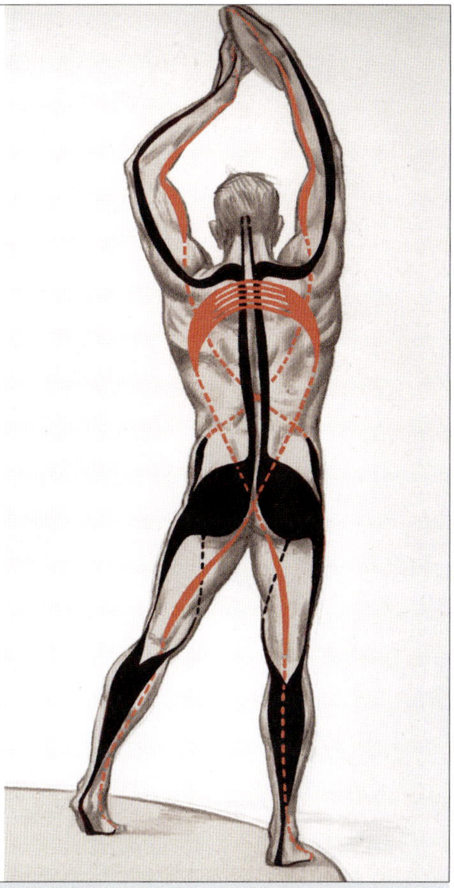

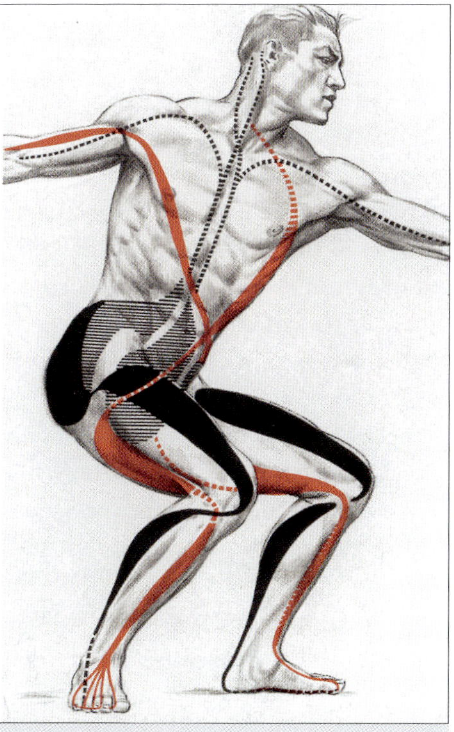

Discus thrower

The throwing performance in track-and-field events is determined by the ability of the athletes to generate a **high degree of final acceleration** in the item of sports equipment by explosive rotational, swinging and streching movements. By "wringing" the upper body against the pelvis, as the discus thrower clearly demonstrates in all three illustrations (fig. 108b), he achieves optimal pre-stretching and a longer acceleration distance, and he brings the maximum acceleration closer to the moment when the discus is released. The **throwing power** which is required for this, is developed above all by the muscles of the trunk, the shoulder joint and the shoulder girdle, and the muscles of the lower extremities. Particular emphasis should be placed on the **interplay between the short and long muscles of the spine and the abdominal muscles,** which are of great importance for throwing.

An increase of muscle mass and power, which is found in a discus thrower and can be seen in the distribution of the two types of muscle fibres (slow-twitch fibres: fast-twitch fibres = 35 % : 65 %), sometimes leads to a **limitation of the mobility of the large joints** (table 16). This is why the stretching capability of the powerful shoulder and hip joint muscles, as well as the mobility of the shoulder girdle, has to be maintained in every training session by means of special exercises.

Table 16: Percentages of slow-twitch fibres (STF) and fast-twitch fibres (FTF) as well as cross-sections (cm^2) of the vastus lateralis of athletes in maximal-power disciplines.

	STF %	FTF %	STF cm^2	FTF cm^2
Weight-lifting	41	59	4550	7430
Discus-throwing	38	62	7200	9580
long jump	45	55	4700	6530
high jump	47	53	6460	7700
100-m sprint	24	76	5400	6750

Muscles Fig. 108b

28 Sternocleidomastoideus
33 Pectoralis major
34 Serratus anterior
35 Obliquus externus abdominis
38 Rectus abdominis
39 Trapezius
42 Latissimus dorsi
44 Teres major
47 Deltoideus
48 Triceps brachii
50 Biceps brachii
51 Brachialis
52 Coracobrachialis
78 Gluteus maximus
79 Gluteus medius
86 Tensor fasciae latae
87 Tractus iliotibialis
89 Gracilis
90 Sartorius
91a Rectus femoris
91b Vastus lateralis
91d Vastus intermedius
94a Biceps femoris, caput longum
94b Biceps femoris, caput breve
96 Semitendinosus
99 Gastrocnemius
100 Soleus
101 Tendo calcaneus
102 Tibialis anterior
103 Extensor digitorum longus
104 Extensor digitorum brevis
107 Fibularis longus
110 Flexor digitorum longus
116 Retinaculum musculorum extensorum superius
117 Retinaculum musculorum extensorum inferius

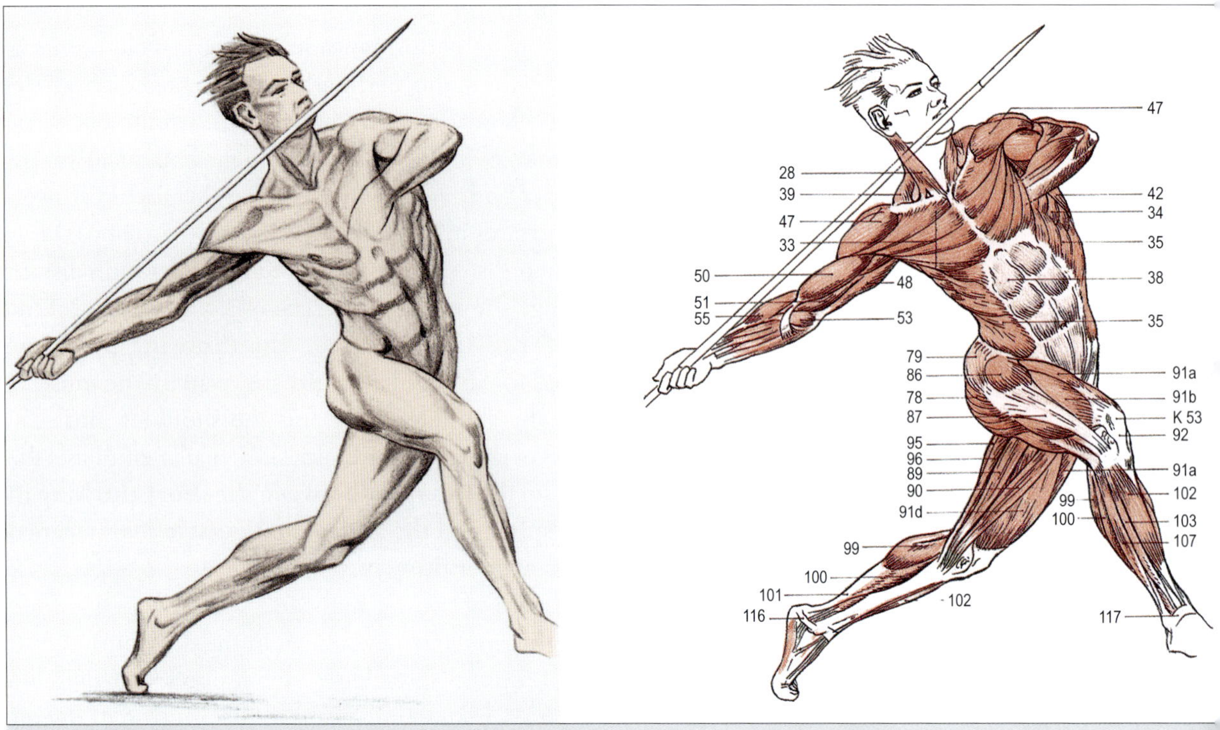

Fig. 109 Muscle slings for the rotation ("wringing") of the trunk in a javelin thrower.

Javelin thrower

After the reader has analysed the sequence of movements of a javelin thrower at the moment of "drawing the bow" of the body (second stage of the releasing phase), up to the moment when the "catapult" of the lower arm is brought into play, he can see in fig. 109 the initial stage which directly precedes the releasing phase with the active muscle slings for **"wringing" the trunk.**

The important point in throwing the javelin is to further increase the speed achieved in the cyclic stage of the running-up phase during the acyclic stage, in order to transfer the **greatest possible accelerative power** to the javelin at the moment of the powerful explosive release.

To achieve this aim great demands are made on the power and coordinative capabilities of the athlete, which apply above all to the optimal technical organization of the release phase. This begins – as shown in the illustrations – with a short and accentuated step; the right leg is then extended in the direction of the throw, while the left leg actively pushes off the track. With the onset of the release phase the final acceleration begins at the moment in which the centre of gravity of the body is above the supporting area of the right leg. At the moment when the left leg, which has been brought forward, touches down, the right hip is brought forward abruptly. This results in an increase of the speed curve. As soon as the left leg has complete contact with the track, the rotating movement around the left foot begins, with the upper body straightening up at the same time ("lifting function" of the left leg), and the second stage of the release (the stage of "drawing the bow" mentioned above) is achieved.

The detailed illustration of the first stage of release emphasizes the point again: throwing the javelin (like all the other throwing and shot track-and-field disciplines) is **a movement of the whole body** and can only be understood and performed successfully with the functional interplay of agonists and antagonists (taking into consideration the set patterns of "closed" linked chains) which are shown in the illustrations of the muscle slings.

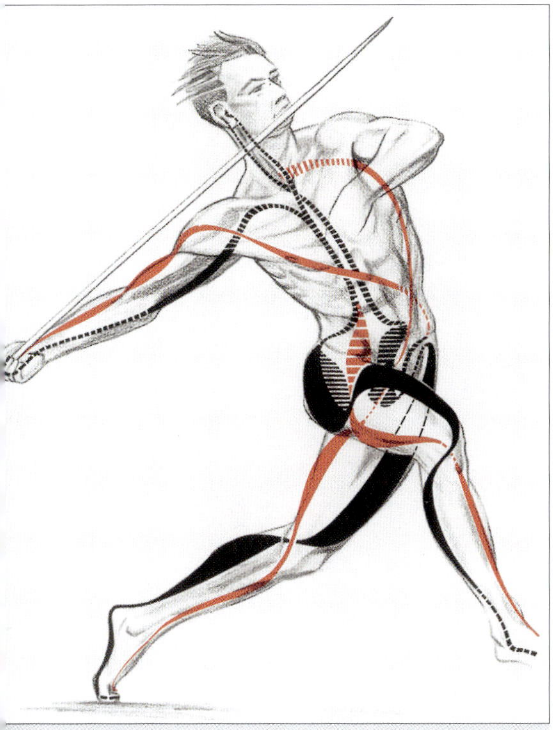

Muscles Fig. 109

28 Sternocleidomastoideus
33 Pectoralis major
34 Serratus anterior
35 Obliquus externus abdominis
38 Rectus abdominis
39 Trapezius
42 Latissimus dorsi
47 Deltoideus
48 Triceps brachii
50 Biceps brachii
51 Brachialis
53 Pronator teres
55 Brachioradialis
78 Gluteus maximus
79 Gluteus medius
86 Tensor fasciae latae
87 Tractus iliotibialis
89 Gracilis
90 Sartorius
91a Rectus femoris
91b Vastus lateralis
91d Vastus intermedius
92 Lig. patellae
95 Semimembranosus
96 Semitendinosus
99 Gastrocnemius
100 Soleus
101 *Tendo* calcaneus
102 Tibialis anterior
103 Extensor digitorum longus
107 Fibularis longus
116 Retinaculum musculorum extensorum superius
117 Retinaculum musculorum extensorum inferius

K53 Patella

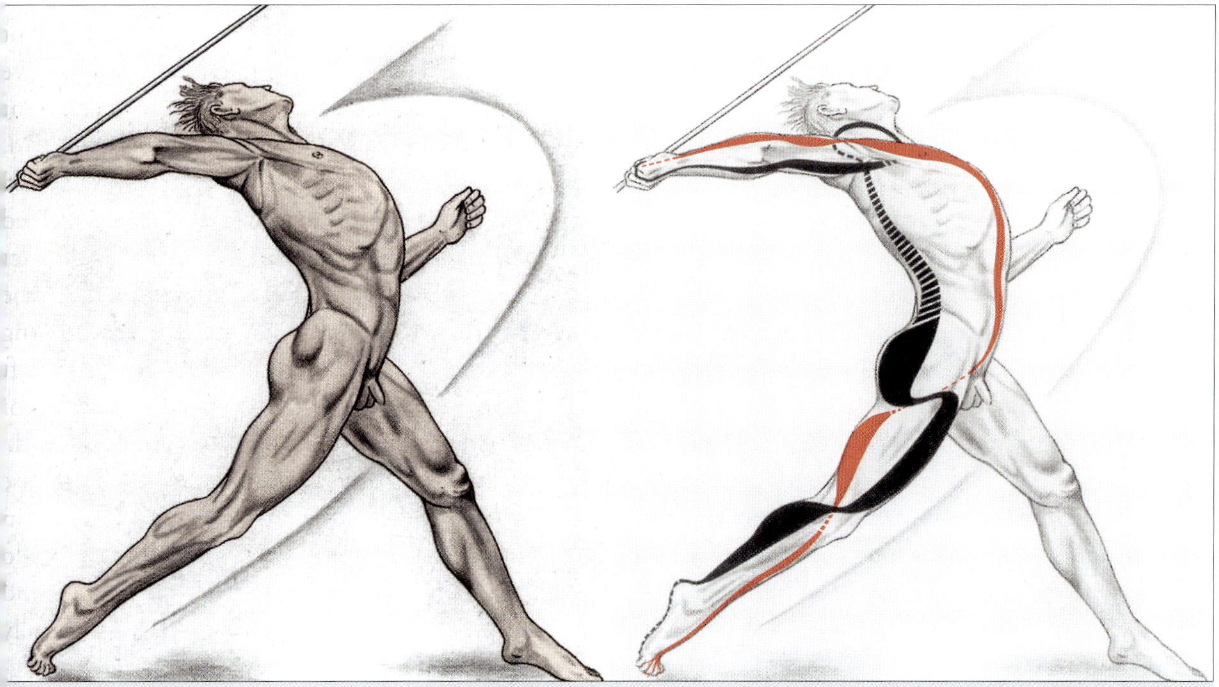

Fig. 110 Javelin thrower at the last moment of "drawing the bow".

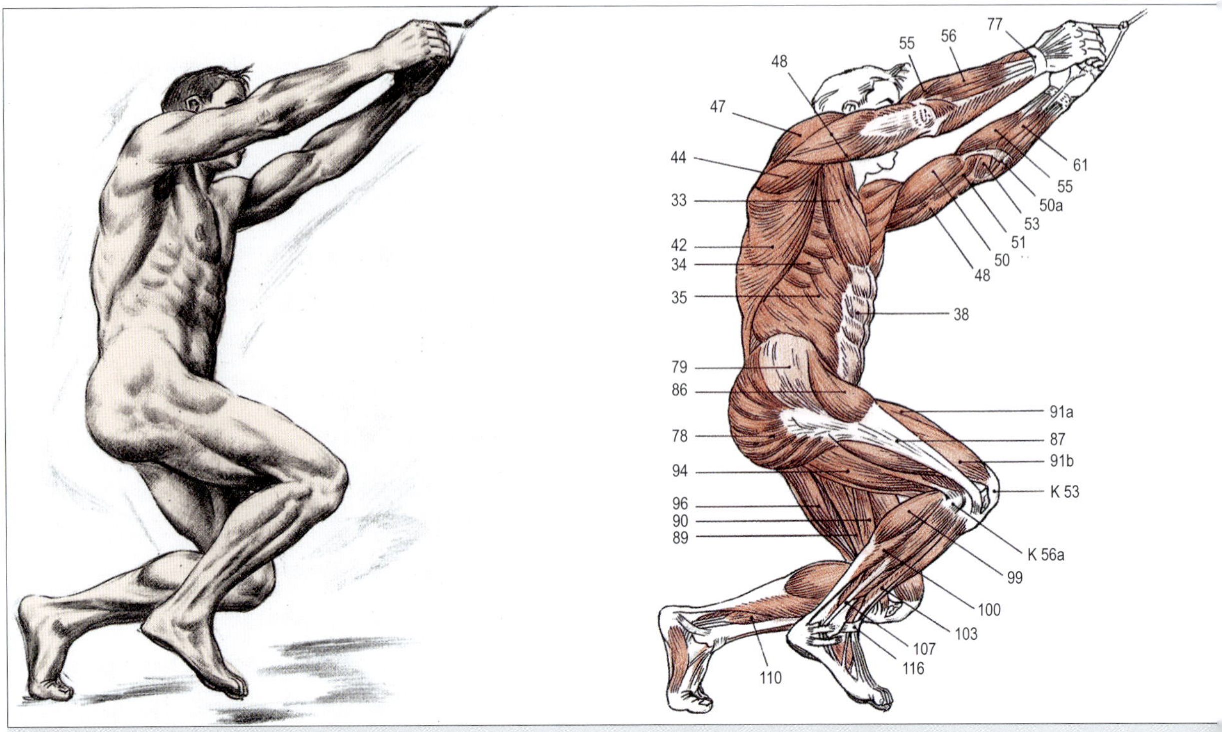

Fig. 111 Muscle slings for the rotation ("wringing") of the trunk in a hammer thrower.

Hammer thrower

This also applies to the next athlete, the hammer thrower (fig. 111), whose discipline is characterized by the complexity of the throwing technique:

- overlapping of 3–4 rhythmical rotational movements during the execution of the throw around varying axes,
- shifts from active accelerative phases – in relation to the 7,25-kg object thrown by men, and 4-kg object thrown by women – to reactive phases, which are distinguished by spatial and postural changes of the body of the athlete in the throwing ring,
- coordination of several partial-body movements,
- great centrifugal force which the thrower has to cope with (which comes to 2450 N in the final phase),
- the transition from rotational movements to the phase of maximal final acceleration, which comes to about 21–23 m/sec.
- the force effect at the handle of the hammer in the direction of the throw of the hammer on the third rotation comes to 4000–4100 N.

In order to master the rotational movements one needs not only technical skills but above all **the capability to develop maximum and rapid power** of all the muscles involved in the sequence of movement, which is shown in the illustration of the slings. In fig. 111, which shows the phase in which the athlete is supporting himself on one leg, particular attention should be paid to the initial (and noticeably increasing) **"wringing" of the trunk to the right** (with the help of the oblique abdominal muscle belt), which is actively supported by the powerful action of the muscles of the left leg and by a rapid turning of the pelvis (both taking place in the direction of the rotation), as well as by the lowering of the left knee joint (by about 5–10 % of the athlete's height) at the start of the rotation on the

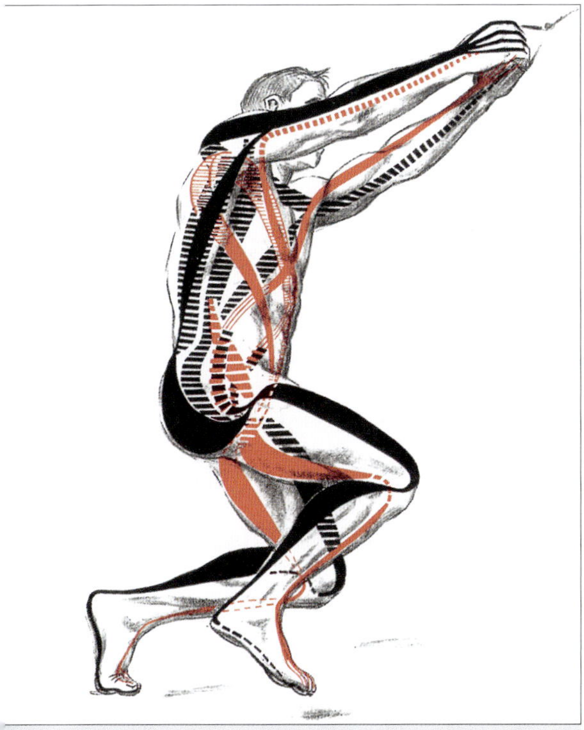

Muscles Fig. 111

33 Pectoralis major
34 Serratus anterior
35 Obliquus externus abdominis
38 Rectus abdominis
42 Latissimus dorsi
44 Teres major
47 Deltoideus
48 Triceps brachii
50 Biceps brachii
50a Aponeurosis bicipitis brachii
51 Brachialis
53 Pronator teres
55 Brachioradialis
56 Extensor carpi radialis longus
61 Flexor carpi radialis
77 Ligg. carpometacarpalia
78 Gluteus maximus
79 Gluteus medius
86 Tensor fasciae latae
87 Tractus iliotibialis
89 Gracilis
90 Sartorius
91a Rectus femoris
91b Vastus lateralis
94 Biceps femoris
96 Semitendinosus
99 Gastrocnemius
100 Soleus
103 Extensor digitorum longus
107 Fibularis longus
110 Flexor digitorum longus
116 Retinaculum musculorum extensorum superius

K53 Patella
K56a Caput fibulae

balls of the foot. This “wringing” of the upper body at the end of the one-leg supporting phase, which reaches its peak at the end of the throw, results in an “overtaking” of the object thrown, if one considers the temporal course of the movement. In this way the necessary precondition for the subsequent acceleration of the object thrown in the next two-leg-support phase is met.

Apart from powerful muscles of the trunk and extensors of the hip, leg and foot, the hammer thrower, who has particularly well-developed muscles, also **requires strong hand and finger flexors** in order to be able to hold the traction load caused by the centrifugal force during the rotations (fig. 112). In addition to maximum and fast-power capabilities, discus and hammer throwers require **great skill and mobility of the shoulder joint and shoulder girdle** and of the lower thoracic and lumbar spine in order to execute throwing movements precisely.

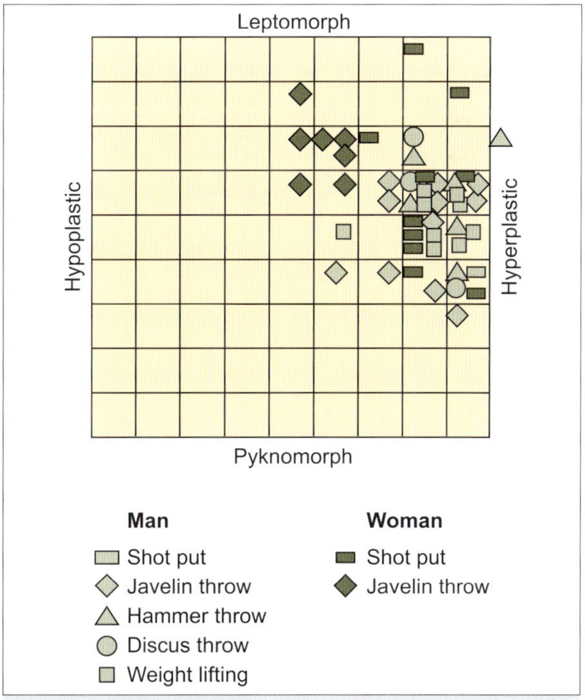

Fig. 112 Distribution of body types in jumping, throwing and lifting disciplines (leptomorph = slender, pyknomorph = overweight, hypoplastic = with underdeveloped muscles, hyperplastic = with prominently developed muscles).

2.7 Combination of muscle slings

Shot-putter

The last sequences of movements are a combination of the now familiar muscle slings and show once again clearly how varied and attractive the interplay of muscles in sport is. This can be seen, among other things, in the active initial phase of a shot-putter (fig. 113), who is of above-average height and weight. The initial phase takes place when the athlete is standing with his or her back facing the direction of the throw in the rear section of the throwing circle, and jumps with his or her right leg. His or her **fast-power capability** – dependent on a proportion of slow- and fast-twitch fibres of 37 % : 63 % – determines above all the extent of the **accelerative impulse,** when the body and arms are fully extended. This impulse, which is the product of the muscles working together synergistically and antagonistically in the slings, is transferred to the shot, which weighs 7,25 kg for men and 4 kg for women, and determines the **shot speed** (14 m/sec is a precondition for shot distances of 22 m and more).

This applies to all the figures shown so far and can be examined with the help of the following investigations. They describe and measure the magnitude of forces that allow the determination of muscular activity by means of electromyography (EMG, see below), accelerometers that enable the quantification of the acceleration of parts of the body, and many other highly technical methods. With the help of these methods the remarkable discovery has been made that the external as well as the internal forces in the joints, tendons and muscles can reach 5–6 times the body force. It is therefore understandable that these great forces are one of the reasons for injuries and stresses in the case of the shot-putter, whose shoulder, trunk, hands and fingers are strongly affected .

Electromyography (EMG) provides an assessment of **intramuscular** coordination during planned movement by helping us to understand

- the size of electrical action potentials, produced by the stimulated muscle cell, whereas the
- EMG amplitude measures the mechanical response to an electrical stimulus.

Simultaneous telemetric EMG recordings from several skeletal muscles during sport-specific movements provide information about the level and duration of the neuronal activity. The development of **intermuscular** coordination can be assessed with this information.

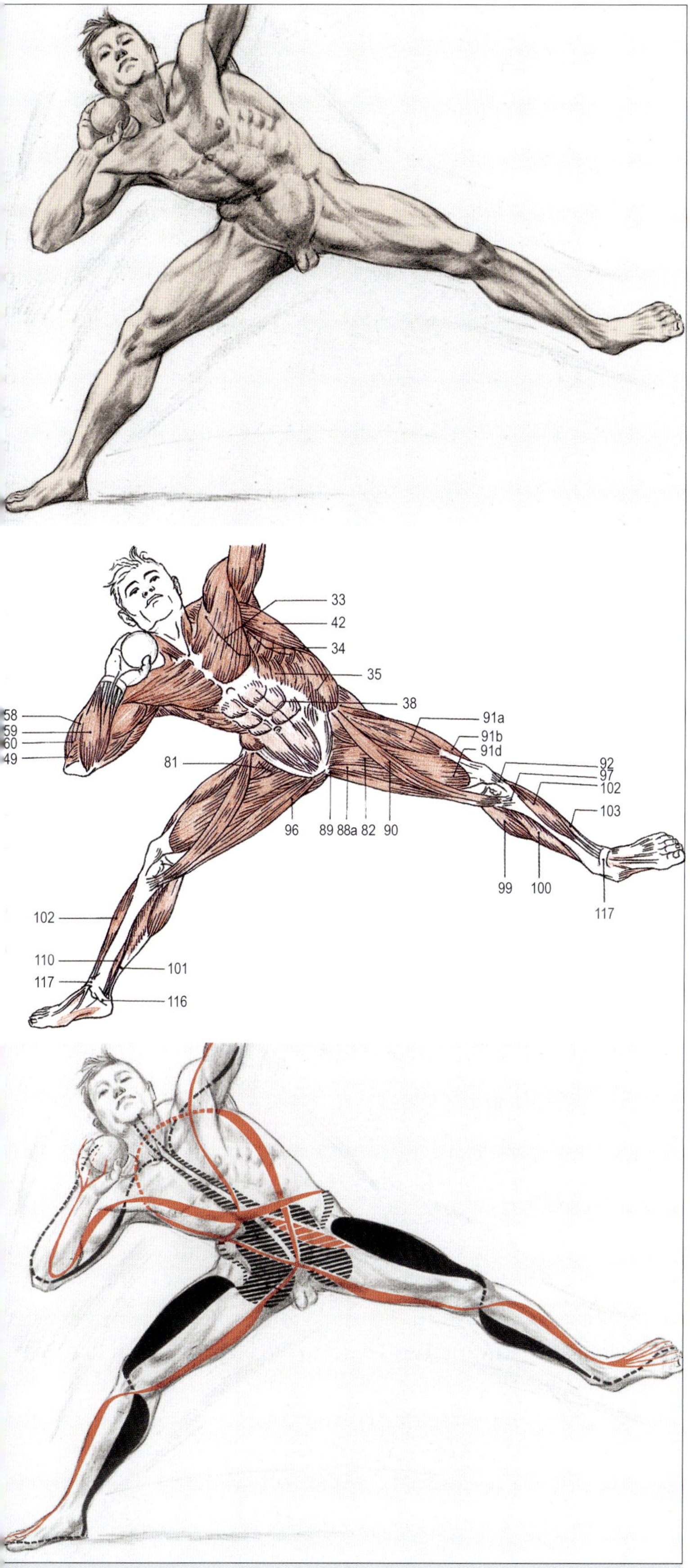

Fig. 113 Combination of muscle slings in a shot-putter.

Muscles Fig. 113

33 Pectoralis major
34 Serratus anterior
35 Obliquus externus abdominis
38 Rectus abdominis
42 Latissimus dorsi
49 Anconeus
58 Extensor carpi ulnaris
59 Flexor carpi ulnaris
60 Extensor digitorum
81 Iliopsoas
82 Pectineus
88a Adductor longus
89 Gracilis
90 Sartorius
91a Rectus femoris
91b Vastus lateralis
91d Vastus intermedius
92 Lig. patellae
96 Semitendinosus
97 Pes anserinus
99 Gastrocnemius
100 Soleus
101 Tendo calcaneus
102 Tibialis anterior
103 Extensor digitorum longus
110 Flexor digitorum longus
116 Retinaculum musculorum extensorum superius
117 Retinaculum musculorum extensorum inferius

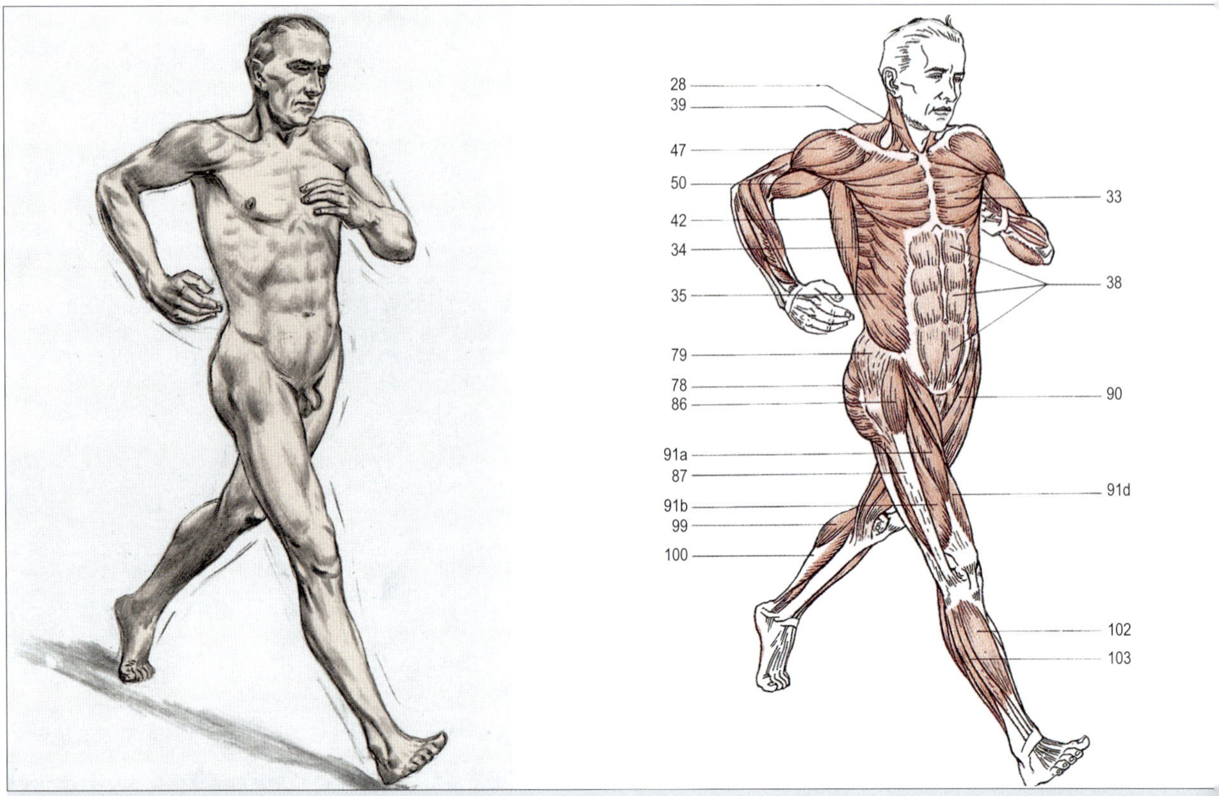

Fig. 114 Combination of muscle slings in a race-walker.

Race-walker

As opposed to normal walking, in race-walking (fig. 114) at a speed of up to 4 m/sec according to the regulations, a double-support phase (duration 0.02 sec) is required as a walking technique, during which **both legs are supposed to have contact with the ground** for a short time, **which necessitates a complete extension at the knee joints** (fig. 115). As opposed to normal walking each step of the race-walker lacks a lifting phase. High-performance walkers have a step frequency of 190/min and a step length of 117 cm over a distance of 20 km (in 50-km-walkers the step frequency is reduced to 188/min and the step length to 110 cm). The step length is sometimes limited by physical characteristics and by the degree of coordinative capabilities. These walkers are distinguished by a well-developed **total-body extensor sling,** which is particulary the case in the lower extremity, as shown in fig. 114. It is supported by the "oblique belt" of the **abdominal muscles** and the **gluteus medius and minimus.** The contraction of these muscles on the side of the standing leg leads to a lifting and rotation of the pelvis, and thus of the hip joint on the opposite side which makes it easy to move the free leg forwards to increase the length of the step and to accelerate the forward movement. This means that an optimal step length requires good mobility at the hip joint and pelvis around the deep axis and the longitudinal axis of the body. The forward movement results from the extension of the hip, knee and upper ankle joints during the support phase, which **brings great stress to bear on the knee joints and its supporting structures** (menisci, lateral and cruciform ligaments). In this context the **fast active movements of the arms,** corresponding to the high step frequency, are striking. The significance of this has already been pointed out in fig. 7 and 29.

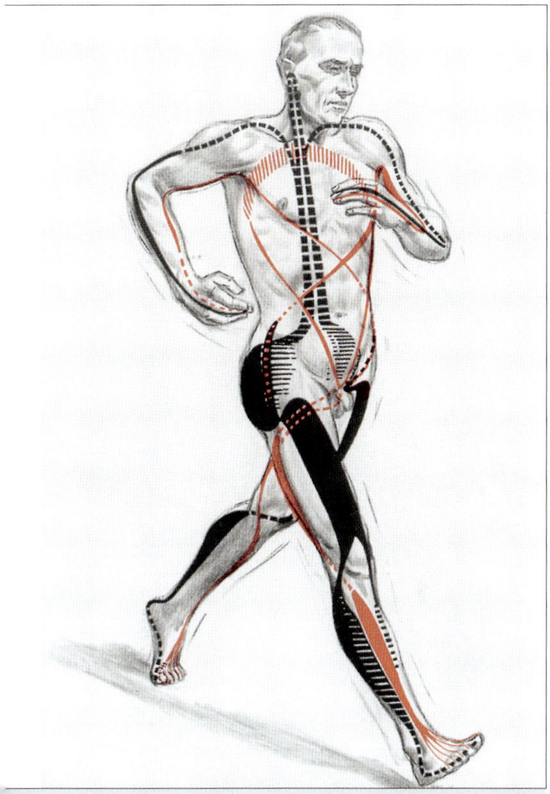

Muscles Fig. 114

28 Sternocleidomastoideus
33 Pectoralis major
34 Serratus anterior
35 Obliquus externus abdominis
38 Rectus abdominis
39 Trapezius
42 Latissimus dorsi
47 Deltoideus
50 Biceps brachii
78 Gluteus maximus
79 Gluteus medius
86 Tensor fasciae latae
87 Tractus iliotibialis
90 Sartorius
91a Rectus femoris
91b Vastus lateralis
91d Vastus intermedius
99 Gastrocnemius
100 Soleus
102 Tibialis anterior
103 Extensor digitorum longus

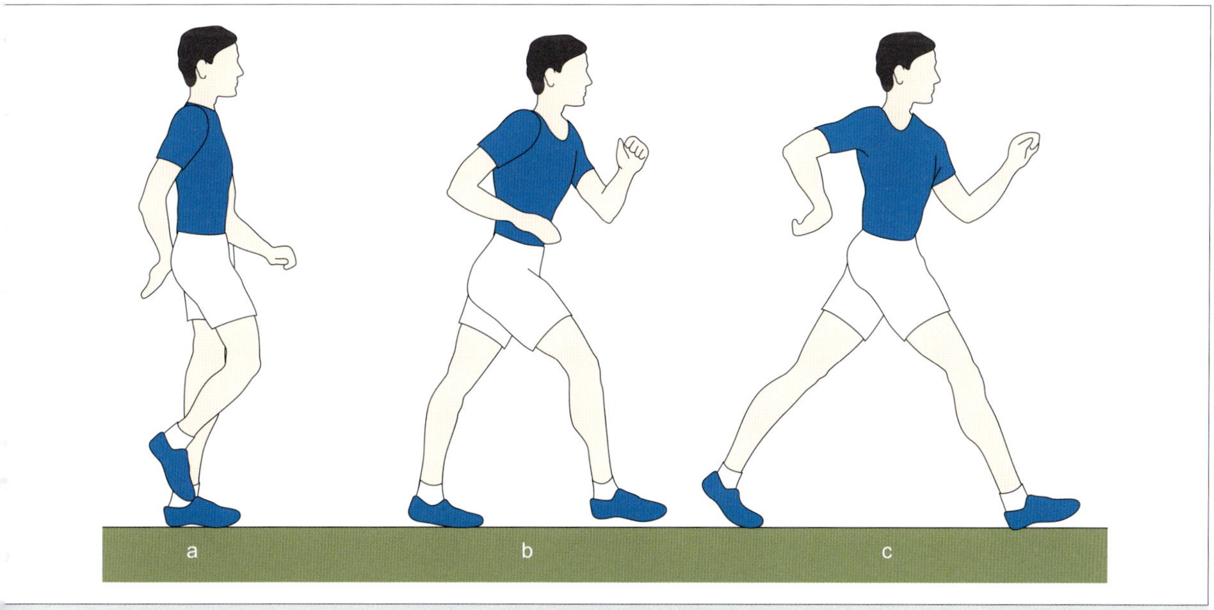

Fig. 115 Race-walking technique for maintaining uninterrupted contact with the ground
a) support phase, b) stretch phase (extreme stretching of the back leg), c) support phase (both feet touching the ground). This demonstrates that the forward swinging leg touches the ground with the heel before the back leg leaves the ground.

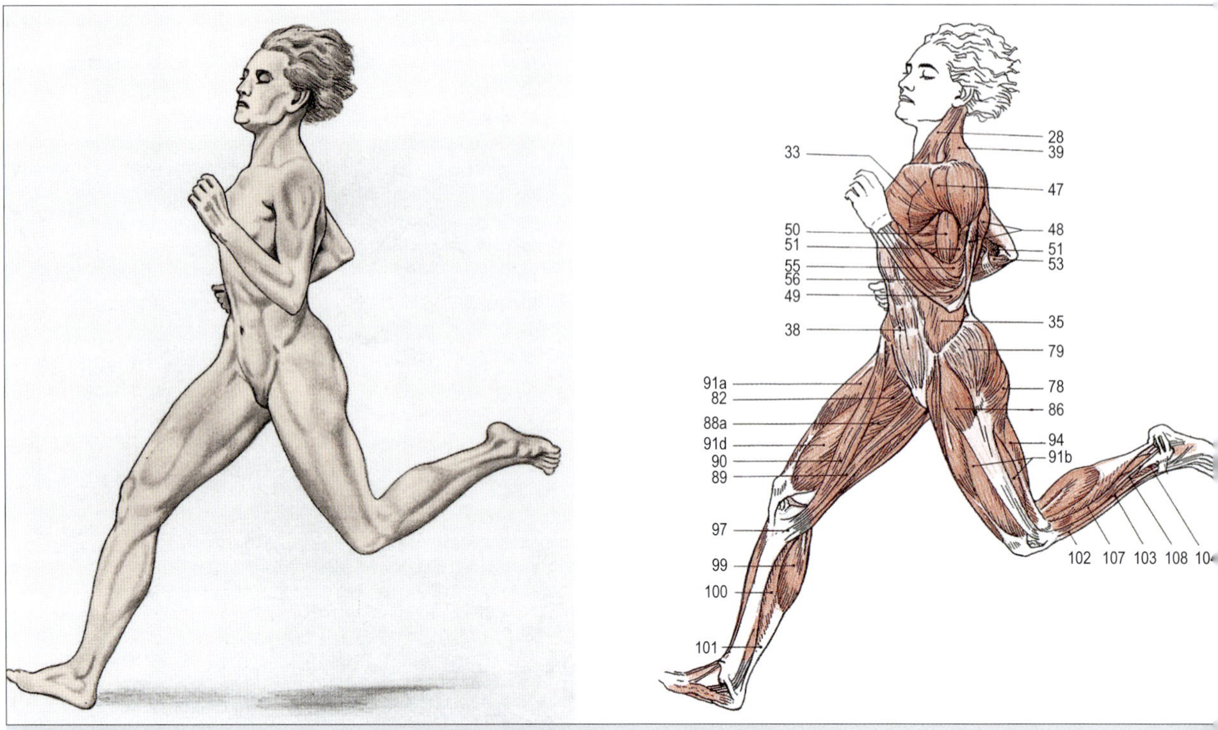

Fig. 116 Combination of muscle slings in a short-distance runner.

Short-distance runner

The final illustration of a short-distance runner (fig. 116) demonstrates once again the cooperation of the muscle slings already mentioned for the extension and "wringing" of the upper body, for the rotation of the pelvis around the vertical axis, in order to increase the step length and acceleration in rhythmic and dynamic walking. It shows that inspite of all the effort involved, sprinting can be an aesthetic type of movement, because the athlete also demonstrates her excellent **coordinative capabilities,** which play a decisive role in successful sports performance along with strength, power, speed and endurance.

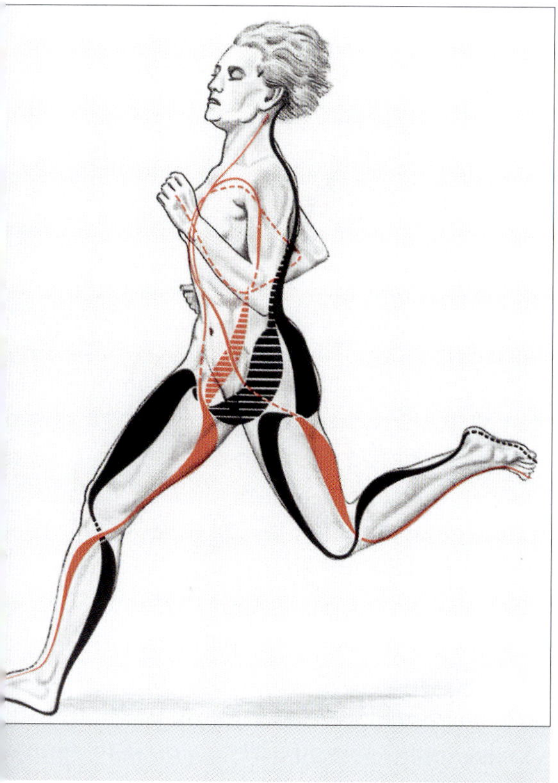

Muscles Fig. 116

- **28** Sternocleidomastoideus
- **33** Pectoralis major
- **35** Obliquus externus abdominis
- **38** Rectus abdominis
- **39** Trapezius
- **47** Deltoideus
- **48** Triceps brachii
- **49** Anconeus
- **50** Biceps brachii
- **51** Brachialis
- **53** Pronator teres
- **55** Brachioradialis
- **56** Extensor carpi radialis longus
- **78** Gluteus maximus
- **79** Gluteus medius
- **82** Pectineus
- **86** Tensor fasciae latae
- **88a** Adductor longus
- **89** Gracilis
- **90** Sartorius
- **91a** Rectus femoris
- **91b** Vastus lateralis
- **91d** Vastus intermedius
- **94** Biceps femoris
- **97** Pes anserinus
- **99** Gastrocnemius
- **100** Soleus
- **101** Tendo calcaneus
- **102** Tibialis anterior
- **103** Extensor digitorum longus
- **104** Extensor digitorum brevis
- **107** Fibularis longus
- **108** Fibularis brevis

Final remarks

Let us therefore make some concluding remarks about the importance of coordination for the muscular balance between synergists and antagonists within the muscle slings.

The early development of motor coordination has many implications for athletes:

- the determination of the limits of the dynamics, efficiency and quality of performance,
- the degree to which the metabolic energy-release mechanisms can be utilized,
- the facilitation of appropriate and rapid responses in the control of body equilibrium to changing situations and conditions,
- the assurance of the performance of certain activities with grace and beauty of movement and
- the protection of competitors from injuries attributable to awkward movements and chronic overloading of muscles, bones and cartilage.

The optimal development of coordinative capabilities serves as a basis for successful **"motor learning"** in every sport and for the performance and the development of sport skills at the highest level. This is particularly important for technical acrobatic sports such as gymnastics, diving and figure skating, as well as for technical events in track-and-field and other sports activities such as running, swimming, wrestling, fencing, boxing and ball games.

From the sports-medical point of view, the coordination of a movement is mainly the internal organization of the optimal control of the motor system and its parts. At stake is the acquisition of motor skills, which can be found in an optimization of the cooperation of motor units in a single muscle (**intramuscular** coordination) or in several muscles (**intermuscular** coordination), including internal or external feedback mechanisms.

The **basis of coordinative capabilities** lies in the highest level of the CNS and sensory motor sub-systems. In the cerebral cortex a motor programme is developed, on the basis of which neuronal impulses are triggered via pyramidal pathways and deeper brain structures, and activate the corresponding skeletal muscles after the motor neuronal pathways have crossed over within the spinal cord. The muscles can thus perform purposeful activities supported by neuronal excitatory and inhibitory processes.

The **training of coordinative capabilities** can be supported during childhood and adolescence by changing the external conditions, which include:

- adjusting boats, lengths and widths of sculls, oars or paddles in accordance with the somato-typical characteristics of rowers and canoeists
- altering the dimensions or adjusting the equipment in gymnastics (e. g. the thickness of the bar)
- reducing the weight of athletic equipment (e. g. of shots, javelins, discs, hammers)
- adjusting ball sizes (handball), ball weights (football) and playing-field sizes.

Appendix

3

Afterword

At the end of this book the reader may in retrospect form his or her own judgment about the extent to which the form of the text and illustrations chosen by the author, for the presentation of movements in sport as a way of making the anatomy lectures for future sports teachers, physio-, sport- and ergotherapists and the continuous education of trainers and sports physicians interesting, are vivid, practical and true-to-life. The **aim** is to make the understanding and learning of the necessary functional-anatomical foundation easier and more meaningful in order to promote the initiative of the individual.
The multifarious muscle interplay is incomprehensible as a unitary performance of our body if one knows only the origin and point of insertion of muscles without their context, but does not understand their different functions in "open" and "closed" muscle slings and the higher functional interrelationships. **The learning and teaching of applied functional-anatomical knowledge** in lectures, seminars, courses and workshops, and not least in textbooks, **must take into account** more than ever **the practical professional needs.**

> *"For those who are not able to see a living person as a transparent body, to visualize the inner form from the surface characteristics and images from memory, anatomy will remain completely lifeless and will not be seen as a tool for active life. But those who learn to see a living person with anatomically trained eyes will discover much that will be revealed to others only through difficult and unreliable technical detours." (Braus, 1960)*

If the reader – with the help of the illustrations – could gain insight into the performance of muscles which take a leading role, with their partners, in the form of **muscle slings** in the sequence of movements, if he or she has got to know the interlinked activity of the individual parts of the motor system, there is still something interesting and worth knowing which remains hidden since the anatomy of a living person is a science with many questions still left open. **Anatomy,** when looked at **from a functional point of view,** increasingly brings together the individual components of our body to form a functional, goal-orientated unity. To demonstrate this with practical examples and to prove it scientifically has been and remains the aim of this book. This has been illustrated by means of numerous sequences of movements in sports, such as track-and-field events, artistic gymnastics, rhythmic gymnastics, dual-combat sports, such as boxing and wrestling, rowing, weight-lifting, and games, such as football and handball. The application of experiments as well as the use of new diagnostic investigations from other scientific disciplines (electromyography, kinematography or video, computer simulation of movement, two- and three-dimensional techniques) will make possible more precise analyses of muscle action in sequences of movements in sport and the application of these results for practical measures to design the content of training in the future.

Source of figures and tables

Figures (also in modified form) and tables, which do not orginate from the author, are taken from the following sources:

3: Kummer, B.: Bauprinzipien des Säugerskeletts. Thieme, Stuttgart 1959

5: Braune, W. u. Fischer, 0.: Der Gang des Menschen, Hirzel, Leipzig 1895

6: Hollmann, W. u. Tittel, K.: Geschichte der deutschen Sportmedizin, 1. Aufl. Druckhaus Gera GmbH 2008

13: Janda, V.: Manuelle Muskelfunktionsdiagnostik. 3. Aufl. Ullstein u. Mosby, Berlin 1994

14: Mollier, G.: Plastische Anatomie, 2. Aufl., Bergmann, München 1938

14, 15, 19: Benninghoff, A.: Lehrbuch der Anatomie des Menschen, Bd. I, 5. Aufl. Urban & Schwarzenberg, Berlin – München 1954; Benninghoff, A. u. Drenckhahn, D.: Anatomie Bd. I, 16. Aufl. Urban & Fischer, München-Jena 2003

20: Waldeyer, A.: Anatomie des Menschen. 6. Aufl. de Gruyter, Berlin 1969

29: Hoepke, H. u. Kantner, M.: Das Muskelspiel des Menschen. 6. Aufl. Fischer, Stuttgart 1971; 7. Auflage 1979

55: Sport Museum (Leipzig, 1968)

Tables 1–11: Lanz, T. u. Wachsmuth, W.: Praktische Anatomie, Bd. 1. Springer, Berlin – Heidelberg – New York 1972

Tables 12–16: eigene Untersuchungen

References

Amtmann, E.: Mechanical stress, functional adaptation and the variation structure of the human femur diaphysis. Ergebn. Anat. Entwick. Gesch. 44/3, 1–89 (1971)

Badtke. G., Ackermann, K. J.: Der Einfluss des Iliosakralgelenks auf die Muskelfunktion und Belastbarkeit des Achsenorgans. Med. Sport 30, 43–44 (1990)

Badtke, G., Bittmann, E., Lazik, D.: Veränderungen der Wirbelsäulenlänge im Tagesverlauf. In: Tittel, K., Arndt, K.-H., Hollmann, W.: Sportmedizin – gestern – heute – morgen. Barth, Leipzig 1993

Baeyer, H.: Die Wirkung der Muskeln auf die menschliche Gliederkette in Theorie und Praxis. Z. Orthop. Chir. 46, 1–19 (1925)

Barrata, R. et al.: Muscular coactivation: The role of the antagonist musculature in maintaining knee stability. Amer. J. Sports Med. 16, 113–122 (1988)

Basmajian, J. V.: Muscles alive. Their functions revealed by electromyography. 5th ed., Williams & Wilkins, Baltimore 1985

Benninghoff, A.: Die Anatomie funktioneller Systeme. Morph. Jb. 65, 1–44 (1931)

Benninghoff, A., Goerttler, K.: Lehrbuch der Anatomie des Menschen, 1. Band: Allgemeine Anatomie, Cytologie und Bewegungsapparat. 11. Auflage, hrsg. und neubearb. von J. Staubesand. Urban & Schwarzenberg, München – Berlin – Wien 1975

Benninghoff, A., Drenckhahn, D.: Anatomie, Bd. 1, 16. Aufl. Urban & Fischer, München – Jena 2003

Berthold, F., Jelinek, W., Albrecht, R.: Die Bedeutung des Muskelfunktionstestes nach Janda für die sportärztliche Praxis. Med. Sport 21, 171–174 (1981)

Beyer, L., Seidel, E. J.: Muskulatur – Funktion und Dysfunktion. Manuelle Medizin 4, 333 (2006)

Braus, A.: Anatomie des Menschen. 1. Band: Bewegungsapparat. 3. Aufl. Springer, Berlin –Göttingen – Heidelberg – New York 1956

Commandre, F.: Appareil locomoteur, sport et société. Med. du Sport 56, 14–16 (1982)

Corvo, R. H.: Morfologia funcional deportiva. Editorial Cientifico-Técnica, Habana 1987

Cotta, H., Krahl, H., Steinbrück, K.: Die Belastungstoleranz des Bewegungsapparates. Thieme, Stuttgart 1980

Daireaux, A., Pottier, M.: Étude électro-myographique de muscles représentatifs du mouvement de l'aviron. Med. du Sport 57, 21–27 (1983)

Dargatz, T.: Fußball-Konditionstraining: Kraft, Schnelligkeit, Ausdauer und Beweglichkeit. Copress Sport, München 2008

Deigentesch, N., Zink, W. und F. Bernett: Die Belastung des Lumbo-Sakralsegments beim Gewichtheben. In: Heck, H. (Hrsg.): Sport: Leistung und Gesundheit. Dtsch. Ärzte-Verlag, Köln 1983

Di Prampero, P. E.: La cout énergétique de la locomotion humaine sur terre et dans l'eau. Schweiz. Zschr. Sportmed. 31, 87–94 (1983)

Engelhardt, M. and A. Dorr (Eds): Sports Orthopedics. Urban & Fischer, München 2012

Faude, 0. et al.: Art und Häufigkeit von Verletzungen im Spitzenfußball der Frauen. Dtsch. Z. Sportmed. 56, 263 (2005)

Fredenhagen, H.: Statik und Dynamik der Wirbelsäule. Schweiz. Zschr. Sportmed. 31, 109–113 (1984)

Fröhner, G.: Haltung und Beweglichkeit des Rumpfes – Merkmale zur Beurteilung der Belastbarkeit. In: Tittel, K., Arndt, K.-H., Hollmann, W.: Sportmedizin – gestern – heute –morgen. Barth, Leipzig 1993

Gregoire, L., Veeger, H.E., Hjuijing, P.A., Van Schenau, G. J.: Role of mono- and biarticular muscles in explosive movements. Int. J. Sports Med. 5, 301–305 (1984)

Groh, H., Baumann, W., Thös, F. R.: Zur Analyse von Bewegungsabläufen im Sport. Sportarzt 17, 392–401 (1966)

Güssbacher, A., Rompe, G.: Die dynamische und statische Beanspruchung der Wirbelsäule und ihre möglichen Auswirkungen bei verschiedenen Sportarten. Schweiz. Zschr. Sportmed. 31, 119–124 (1983)

Gutberlett, I.: Einfluss des sportartspezifischen Trainings auf die arthromuskulären Bezie- hungen und die Belastbarkeit des Stütz- und Bewegungssystems. In: Tittel, K., Arndt, K.-H., Hollmamnn, W. (Hrsg.): Sportmedizin – gestern – heute – morgen. Barth, Leipzig 1993

Hebestreit, H.: Die Mechanik des menschlichen Körpers beim beidarmigen Gewichtdrücken und beidarmigen Gewichtreißen. Pflüg. Arch. 234, 437 (1934)

Heitkamp. H.-C., Mayer, F., Böhm, S.: Effekte eines Klettertrainings im Vergleich zum isometrischen Krafttraining auf die wirbelsäulenstabilisierende Muskulatur. Säule 10,1,26–31 (2000)

Hochschild, J.: Strukturen und Funktionen begreifen – Funktionelle Anatomie – Therapierelevante Details. Thieme, Stuttgart – New York 2002

Hoepke, H. u. Kantner, M.: Das Muskelspiel des Menschen. 6. Aufl. Fischer, Stuttgart 1971; 7. Auflage 1979

Hoppeler, H.: Exercise-induced ultrastructural changes in skeletal muscle. Int. J. Sports Med. 7, 187–204 (1986)

Janda, V.: Manuelle Muskelfunktionsdiagnostik, 3. Aufl. Ullstein Mosby, Berlin 1994

Junge, A. et al.: Verletzungen beim Handball, Fußball und Basketball während der Olympischen Spiele 2004 in Athen. Dtsch. Z. Sportmed. 56, 263 (2005)

Kapandji. I. A.: Funktionelle Anatomie der Gelenke. 3. Aufl. Hippokrates-Verlag, Stuttgart 1999

Kjaer, M.: Anpassung der Sehnen an körperliche Belastung. Dtsch. Z. Sportmed. 55, 6, 148–151 (2004)

Klein, P., Sommerfeld, P.: Biomechanik der menschlichen Gelenke. Urban & Fischer, München – Jena 2004

Klein, P., Sommerfeld, P.: Biomechanik der Wirbelsäule. Urban & Fischer, München – Jena 2007

Komi, P. V, Häkkinen, K.: Strength and power. In: Dirix, A., Knuttgen, H. G., Tittel. K. (Eds.): Olympic Book of Sports Medicine, pp. 181–193. Blackwell, Oxford 1989

Krämer, J.: Praktische Konsequenzen zur Belastbarkeit der Wirbelsäule beim Sport. Prakt. Orthop. Bd. 7, 41–44 (1977)

Kummer, B.: Die Biomechanik der aufrechten Haltung. Mitt. d. Naturf. Ges. Bern, Bd. 22 (1965)

Lanz, T., Wachsmuth, W.: Praktische Anatomie. Bd. 1. Springer, Berlin – Heidelberg – New York, 1972

Larsson, L.: Morphological muscle characteristics in rowers. Can. J. Appl. Sport Sci. 5, 239–244 (1980)

Lèbe-Néron, R. M., Perron, G.: La représentation du mouvement humain par ordinateur. Science and Sports 3, 303–313 (1988)

Lephart, S. et al.: Gender differences in strength and lower extremity kinematics during landing. Clin. Orthop. Rel. Res. 401, 162–169 (2002)

Lippert, H.: Lehrbuch Anatomie. 5. Aufl. Urban & Fischer, München – Jena 2000

MacConaill, M. A., Basmajian, J. V.: Muscles and Movements – a Basis for Human Kinesiology. Williams & Wilkins, Baltimore 1969

Miller, D. J.: Ground reaction forces in distance running. Champaign 203–224 (1990)

Mollier, S.: Plastische Anatomie. 2. Aufl. Bergmann, München 1938

Moore, M. A., Hutton, R. S.: Electromyographic investigation of muscle stretching technique. Med. Sci. Sports Exerc. 12, 322–329 (1980)

Münchinger, R.: Die auf die Wirbelsäule wirkenden mechanischen Kräfte. Formen und Haltungen der Wirbelsäule. Huber, Bern 1964

Neumann, G., Buhl, H.: Biologische Leistungsvoraussetzungen und trainings-physiologische Aspekte bei trainierenden Frauen. Med. Sport 21, 154–160 (1981)

Neumann, G., Berbalk, A.: Sport- und Wettkampftauglichkeit bei Langzeitausdauerbelastungen. Med. Sport 28, 161–167 (1988)

Neumann, G., Schüler, K.-P.: Sportmedizinische Funktionsdiagnostik. 2. Aufl. Barth, Leipzig 1994

Pauwels, F.: Gesammelte Abhandlungen zur funktionellen Anatomie des Bewegungsapparates. Springer, Berlin – Heidelberg – New York 1965

Riepenhausen, U., Lachmann, D.: Zum Einsatz des Janda-Testes für die Objektivierung muskulärer Dysbalancen und deren Beseitigung durch Bewegungstherapie in der Sportmedizin. Z. Physiother. 36, 53–57 (1984)

Scherb, R.: Kinematisch-diagnostische Analyse von Gangstörungen, Technik und Resultate der Myokinesigraphie. Enke, Stuttgart 1952

Schmidt, H. et al.: Der Muskelfunktionstest nach Janda für die sportmedizinische Praxis. Med. Sport 23, 271–278 (1983)

Schnabel, G., Harre, D., Krug, J., Borde, A.: Trainingswissenschaft. 3. Aufl. Sportverlag, Berlin 2002

Silvers, H. K., Mandelbaum, B. R.: Prevention of anterior cruciate ligament injury in the female athlete. Br. J. Sports Med. 41, 52–59 (2007)

Solomonow, M. et al.: The synergistic action of the anterior cruciate ligament and thigh muscles in maintaining joint stability. Amer. J. Sports Med. 15 (1987), 207–213

Solomonow, M., Krogsgaard, M.: Sensorimotor control of knee stability. Scand J. Med. Sci. Sports 11, 64–80 (2001)

Stehle, P.: Biomechanische Belastungsuntersuchungen an mehrbelasteten Röhrenknochen. In: Tittel, K., Arndt, K.-H., Hollmann, W.: Sportmedizin – gestern – heute – morgen. Barth, Leipzig 1993

Steinacker, J. M.: Physiological aspects of training in rowing. Int. J. Sports Med. 14 (1993), 3–10

Thom, H.: Elektromyographische Funktions-Analyse der Schulter- und Armmuskulatur. Verh. dtsch. Orthop. Ges. 1964

Thorstensson, A.: Speed and acceleration. In: Dirix, A., Knuttgen, H.G., Tittel, K.: Olympic Book of Sports Medicine, pp. 218–229. Blackwell, Oxford 1989

Tittel, K.: Zur Entwicklung der funktionellen Betrachtungsweise in der Anatomie. Festvortrag anlässlich Literaturpreis-Verleihung 1963. Theor. u. Prax. Körperkult. 9 (1963)

Tittel, K.: Zur Biotypologie und funktionellen Anatomie des Leistungssportlers. Barth, Leipzig –Berlin – Heidelberg 1965

Tittel, K., Wutscherk, H.: Sportanthropometrie. Barth, Leipzig-Berlin-Heidelberg 1972

Tittel, K.: The influence of work load of different duration and intensity on hypertrophy, pulling stability and extension capacity of dense collagen connective tissue. Brit. J. Sportsmed. 78–84 (1973)

Tittel, K.: Funktionelle Anatomie und Biomechanik des Kniegelenks. Med. u. Sport 17, 65–72 (1977)

Tittel, K.: Die Belastbarkeit der Wirbelsäule unter Berücksichtigung funktionell-anatomischer und biomechanischer Gesichtspunkte. Med. u Sport 21, 3–10 (1981)

Tittel, K.: Functional anatomy of the spine. Medisport 3, 8, 248–256 (1981)

Tittel, K.: Morphologische Grundlagen für die Funktionsdiagnostik des Bewegungsapparates. Z. Physiother. 36, 11 (1984)

Tittel, K.: Bewegungsabläufe in der Leichtathletik unter dem Gesichtspunkt der Muskelschlingen. In: Kurz, D., Schütte, U.: Leichtathletik. Hofmann, Schorndorf 1986

Tittel, K.: Funktionell-anatomische und biomechanische Grundlagen für die Sicherung des arthromuskulären Gleichgewichts im Sport –ein Beitrag zur Erhöhung der Belastbarkeit bindegewebiger Strukturen. Med. Sport 26, 2–4 (1986)

Tittel, K.: Functional-anatomical and biomechanical fundamentals for safeguarding the arthro-muscular balance in sports. In: Mácek, M., Kucera, M. : Sports in health and disease. Avicenum Med. Press, Prague 1987

Tittel, K.: Coordination and Balance. In: Dirix, A., Knuttgen, H. G., Tittel, K.: Olympic Book of Sports Medicine, pp. 194–211. Blackwell, Oxford 1989

Tittel, K.: Età evolutiva ed adattamenti della forza del muscolo scheletrico. L'esempio del sollevamento pesi. Rivista di cultura sportiva 19, 22–30 (1990)

Tittel, K., Wutscherk, H.: Anatomical and anthropometric fundamentals of endurance. Vol. II. Olympic Book of Sports Medicine, pp. 35–45. Blackwell, Oxford 1992

Tittel, K., Wutscherk, H.: Biological basis for strength and power – anthropometric factors. Vol. III. Olympic Book of Sports Medicine, pp. 180–196. Blackwell, Oxford 1992

Tittel, K.: Funktionelle Anatomie und Biomechanik der Sprunggelenke. TW Sport + Medizin 9, 4,172–178 (1997)

Tittel, K.: Funktionell-anatomische und biomechanische Aspekte der Lenden-Hüftregion und ihrer Belastung. Die Säule 8, 4, 14–19 (1998)

Tittel, K.: Funktionelle Anatomie im Sport –Historisch-systematische Facetten. Akademie-Verlag, Sankt Austin 2002

Tittel, K.: Anatomia descritiva e funcional do corpo humano. Livraria Santos Editora 2006

Tittel, K.: Kreuzband-Verletzungen im Frauen-Fußball – Ursachen und Mechanismen aus funktionell-anatomischer Sicht. Ref. FIFA-Fußball-WM der Frauen. Dresden 2011

Tittel, K., Seidel, E. J.: Beschreibende und funktionelle Anatomie. 15. Aufl., Kiener, München 2012

Vandervael, F.: Analyse des mouvements du corps humain. Librairie Maloine et Editions Desoer, Paris – Liège (1951)

Viel, E.: Bioméchanique de l'épaule et incidences sur la rééducation. Med. du Sport 54, 49–55 (1980)

Williams, K. R., Cavanagh, P. R.: Relationship between distance running mechanics, running economy and performance. J. Appl. Physiol. 63, 1236–1245 (1987)

Wirhed, R.: Sport-Anatomie und Bewegungslehre. Schattauer, Stuttgart – New York 1984

Wittekopf, G., Rühl, H.: Beispiele oberflächen-elektromyographischer Untersuchungen zur Beurteilung der muskulären Koordination sportlicher Bewegungsabläufe. Med. Sport 24, 229–232 (1984)

Zatsiorski, V. M.: Krafttraining – Praxis und Wissenschaft. Meyer & Meyer, Aachen 1996

Index

(**bold** page numbers refer to figures; authors mentioned in *italic*)

A

B

F

G

H

I

M

N

O

P

Q

R

S

T

U

V

W